EVERYTHING YOU NEED TO KNOW ABOUT CAREGIVING FOR PARKINSON'S DISEASE

EVERYTHING YOU NEED TO KNOW ABOUT CAREGIVING FOR PARKINSON'S DISEASE

The Complete Guide for Anyone Caring for Someone with Parkinson's Disease

LIANNA MARIE

It is not the purpose of this publication to reprint all the information that is otherwise available about Parkinson's disease, but to compliment, amplify, and supplement other sources of information. You should NOT rely solely upon the information, content or opinions within this publication.

Rather, you are urged to read all the available material, learn as much as possible about Parkinson's disease, and tailor the information to your individual needs.

Every effort has been made to make the information contained herein as accurate as possible. Also note that although this publication is updated often, medical information changes rapidly. Therefore, please be advised some information may be out of date and there may be errors, both typographical and in content. Therefore, this publication should only be used as a general guide, and not as the ultimate source of Parkinson's disease information.

The information in this publication is provided for educational and informational purposes only, and is not intended to be a substitute for a health care provider's consultation. Please consult your own physician or appropriate health care provider about the applicability of any opinions or recommendations with respect to your own symptoms or medical conditions.

Always consult with your physician or other qualified health care provider before embarking on a new treatment, diet, or fitness program. You should never disregard medical advice or delay in seeking it because of something you have read in this publication.

The Author, Publisher, and any contributing parties specifically disclaim any liability, loss, or risk that is incurred as a consequence, directly or indirectly, of the use and application of any contents of this work.

To Dave.

For all that you meant to us, the Parkinson's world, and especially to Mom, we thank you with all our hearts. Even until the very end, you cared most about her well-being and not your own.

To Mom.

Thank you for helping me become a better daughter and caregiver throughout this journey with you. I love you so much and would go to the moon and back to give you the quality of life you want and deserve.

TABLE OF CONTENTS

--- ~ ---

Acknowledgements

--- ~ ---

I wish to thank the following people for their
generous support and belief in this project:

Nick Badran

Kathi Ballou

Barbara J. Brady

Arnold Biscontini

David and Vinnice Blow

Elvira Brunt

Maxine Cable

Charles Chen

David Dameron

Tim Doherty

Tanya Galloway

Rebecca Jo JamesCourie

Ronald D. Jones

Muriel Lehto

Jean-Yves Leon

Timothy L. McGuirk

Kenneth V. Mutlow

Dr. Dominic Noonan

Claire nyiti

Denise C. Pelkey

Judy Recher

Robert L. Sharkey

Tina Shipman

Joanne Stuffel

Susan Timmins

Vicki Warren

Craig Werner

Penny Wigglesworth

--- ~ ---

--- ~ ---
Why I Wrote this Book
--- ~ ---

My mom has Parkinson's and dementia. She has been in the Parkinson's "battle" for over 25 years and the dementia one for about three.

I think most would say that it's pretty remarkable Mom has made it this far in her journey with Parkinson's, given that the average time people with this disease have from diagnosis to death is 16 years.

I believe it's been her faith and determination, as well as the caregivers she's had over the years, that have made the biggest difference.

Mom's been fortunate enough to have a team of people around her that helped make life easier as her illness progressed. In the early stages of her disease, she married Dave (my step-dad), and he took on the role of primary caregiver.

Though initially Dave's caregiving duties consisted of helping with simple tasks like assisting Mom out of a chair now and then, over time these duties became more and more involved.

Tasks like helping her walk to the bathroom when Mom's wheels (a.k.a. legs) were shut down, delivering medications to her at the scheduled times, and taking on household jobs like cooking and cleaning were just a few of the things that Dave took on. He also took charge of trying to maintain a stress-free environment for Mom so as to minimize her symptoms – an assignment most people would find challenging.

As the years passed, the physical stress and emotional demands of caregiving became too much for Dave, so both he and my mom sought external help. This help took many forms, including care workers who helped them in their home, support groups for both of them, short-term respite from a care facility, and caregiving from family members like myself.

Unfortunately, throughout his many years of caring for Mom, Dave neglected to take care of himself. He developed diabetes and was later diagnosed with two separate types of cancer.

Despite his illnesses, Dave was a loyal and loving caregiver. He visited Mom in the nursing home and took her on outings whenever he was able. He even volunteered and helped raise funds for his local Parkinson's foundation.

Sadly, his illnesses became too much for him, and one late June evening two years ago, Dave passed away.

I know our story is not unique. Having read hundreds of stories from fellow Parkinson's caregivers, I found that many are doing their utmost for their loved ones with Parkinson's, but are finding it overwhelming and sometimes detrimental to their own health.

As a long-distance caregiver and advocate for my mom, I have embarked upon a mission to help her receive the best quality and quantity of care possible. After seeing the toll that caregiving took on Dave, but conversely what his and my family's efforts have done to help improve Mom's quality of life, I feel compelled to help other caregivers care for themselves while caring for their loved ones.

My hope is that this book can be the beginning of a new chapter in your caregiving journey – one in which you find encouragement and support, as well as practical tips and guidance to help you navigate the various challenges you may face.

I will finish with a quote from an interview Mom gave around the 12th year of her journey with Parkinson's. She was speaking about what enabled her to keep going day after day, but I think it applies to us caregivers as well.

Each day we must remind ourselves *why* we do what we do. We must find meaning in our lives outside of caregiving and focus on the joys and fulfillment we can gain from caring for our loved one.

"You have to feel that there is a purpose for you getting up today, that there is something meaningful for you to do. That it's not going to be the same ol' battle." ~ Mom

--- ~ ---

--- ~ ---

PART 1
CAREGIVING 101

--- ~ ---

CHAPTER 1
Who Cares?

Never believe that a few caring people can't change the world.
For, indeed, that's all who ever have.
~ Margaret Mead

Merriam-Webster defines a caregiver as a "person who gives help and protection to someone (such as a child, an old person, or someone who is sick)". In this book we will be discussing issues specific to those caring for someone with Parkinson's disease, and also issues that are relevant to caregivers of any kind.

Yes, it's important that you understand that regardless of whom you are caring for, many of the issues you will face are relevant to ALL caregivers. In other words, you are not alone.

In fact, you may be surprised to learn just how many caregivers there are in this world. Estimates say there are almost 44 million people providing care for a family member or loved one in the United States, 8.1 million in Canada, 6.5 million in the UK, and 2.7 million in Australia... And those are just the countries on which we could find statistics!

Caregiving can be a very rewarding job; in fact, a 2014 survey from the National Opinion Research Center in the US found that 83 percent of caregivers view it as a positive experience.

Many say they like the positive experience they get from giving something back to someone who cared for them, as well as the satisfaction of knowing that their loved one is getting the quality of care they want. Caregivers also report they feel that taking care of their loved one gives them purpose in their lives.

Unfortunately, on the flip side, many caregivers are incredibly overworked, stressed out, or depressed. Whether you care for someone with Parkinson's or dementia, or simply an aging parent, caregiving can take huge tolls on your health and finances if you're not careful.

Here are some quick stats on Caregiving in the US:
(All stats taken from a 2015 report done by the American
Association of Retired Persons - "AARP")

- Nearly 44 million adults in the US are providing personal assistance for family members with disabilities or other care needs.
- Six in 10 caregivers are female.
- The average age of caregivers in the US is 49.
- The typical caregiver has been helping a parent or spouse for four years.
- More than 15 million caregivers provide care for someone with dementia.
- A third of family caregivers say they do it alone, receiving no help from anyone.
- Over one quarter of caregivers are "sandwiched" between caregiving and raising children.
- Six in 10 caregivers care for an adult with a long-term physical condition.
- Six in 10 caregivers are employed.
- Fifty percent of caregivers feel they had no choice in choosing their caregiver role.

CHAPTER 2
Types of Caregivers

Family is not an important thing. It's everything.
~ Michael J. Fox

There are many types of caregivers; some live in the same house as their loved one, whereas others live miles and miles away. Some are spouses, while others are sons or daughters. Some may even care for a parent while still caring for their own children.

Caregiving can entail a myriad (as in, a LOT!) of things, including helping with house cleaning, doctor's appointments, or finances, or it can be more "hands on," like helping your loved one with getting dressed, bathing, and/or going to the bathroom.

I have been my mom's caregiver, both in a live-in situation and living far away from her.

The following are the main types of caregivers to whom most organizations refer. Note that you may fall into more than one of these categories:

The Crisis Caregiver - This term applies if your loved one or family member does fine on his or her own until there's an emergency - that's when you step in.

The Working Caregiver - You are taking on a caregiving role (be it physical and/or financial) in addition to holding down a part-time or full-time job.

The Sandwich Caregiver - This term was coined to describe those caregivers who take care of not only their children, but their elderly parents too. They are "sandwiched" between two generations.

The Spousal Caregiver - When a life partner becomes ill, a caregiver must deal with many challenging and sometimes heart-wrenching issues, including adjusting to one's partner becoming the patient, as well as intimacy issues.

The Long-Distance Caregiver - If you live in a different city, state/province, or country, you are a long-distance caregiver. Despite the fact that they live far away, long-distance caregivers can be responsible for the financial, medical, and personal needs of their loved ones and help them by telephone.

CHAPTER 3
Before You Say "Yes" to Caregiving

We know what we are, but know not what we may be.
~ William Shakespeare

Caregiving is a choice. Though as many as half of all caregivers say they never chose their caregiving gig, you need to know that whether or not you *feel* you have a choice, you really do.

Before blindly rushing into caregiving, it's a good idea to look at your own physical, emotional, and financial needs first.

Here are three important questions you should answer honestly before you take steps into the caregiving world:

1. Are you physically and emotionally ready?

Most people who take on the caregiving role aren't prepared for its many challenges and how quickly it takes over your life.

The good news is you *can* make the caregiving journey a more pleasant and rewarding one by readying yourself ahead of time. How? A key factor is to become empowered. Tell yourself you can do this! Face your fears of "not being qualified for the job" and break free of beliefs that may be limiting you.

Another thing you'll want to think about as you contemplate taking on the caregiving role is how it will affect your relationships. If you are married, is your spouse supportive of or negative towards caregiving? If you don't have a spouse, how will this affect your ability to be a caregiver? If you have kids, how will your caregiver role affect them and your relationship with them?

2. Are you financially ready?

Caring for a family member can carry a heavy price tag and make a serious impact on a caregiver's personal finances. As we will discuss in a later chapter, it's imperative that you plan your finances ahead of time. Additional factors such as whether or not you have children and the state of your care-receiver's finances will also impact your decision as to whether or not you'll take on the caregiving role.

3. Are you legally ready?

Do you know your loved one's wishes in the end stages of their life? Do they have a plan to pay for their care if needed? Without certain legal documents in place, caring for your loved one can be a lot more difficult than it needs to be.

You can help your loved one plan for their current and future medical and financial needs by working with them to prepare six essential legal documents. You can read more about these in Chapter 7, "Making a Plan".

Having the necessary documents in order before a medical or financial disaster strikes can make an extremely difficult situation just a little bit easier to navigate.

In addition, knowing that you're carrying out your loved one's wishes can give you valuable peace of mind and ease feelings of guilt that many caregivers experience in these situations.

Can I say "No" to Caregiving?

Maybe you've taken an honest look at your ability and willingness to commit to being a caregiver and are feeling that it's not right for you. If that's the case and you're looking for permission to say "no" to caregiving, no one is going to give it to you – except you.

You may think, 'But I can't say 'no' to Mom. She was always there for me growing up; how could I NOT be there for her now?" Rest easy;

caregiving isn't for everyone. Though it's tough saying "no" to your loved one, sometimes it's actually the less selfish, more loving, and more caring thing to do.

Passing the role onto another family member or professional can save you from burning out and may even strengthen your relationship with your loved one if done with love and honesty.

In my case, I don't know if there was ever a question as to whether or not I would care for my mom – it was more a question of how I could *best* care for her.

In the beginning I learned that supporting my stepdad (Mom's primary caregiver at the time) was the best way for me to care for her. Then, as her care needs became greater and it became apparent that my stepdad was getting burned out, I became more involved in Mom's care.

Years later, my family (in consultation with my Mom and stepdad) made the decision to move her to a care facility. This helped take the burden off all of us while allowing her to get the care she needed. I don't consider this to have been us saying "no" to caregiving, but rather making a choice to care for her in a different way.

There is no right or wrong when it comes to the decision of caregiving. Everyone is different and you have to make the choices that are best for you.

--- ~ ---

PART 2
WHAT TO EXPECT

--- ~ ---

CHAPTER 4
After You've Said "Yes" to Caregiving

From caring comes courage.
~ Lao Tzu

Life with Parkinson's is unpredictable. Once you've decided to take on the role of caregiver, it's important that you learn how to plan ahead and be ready to adapt to changes in your loved one's health and care needs.

Planning ahead is also essential so you don't undermine your own health while caring for your loved one.

Here are four key things you'll want to do after you've decided to say "yes" to caregiving:

1. Get organized

When it comes to caring for people with Parkinson's, the importance of getting organized and planning ahead cannot be overemphasized. Without the right legal and financial documentation, you and your loved one could face many problems in an emergency.

Doctors may refuse to discuss important medical information with you, and your loved one may not get the end-of-life care they desire. Also, if your loved one becomes incapacitated, control over their bank accounts and property could be given to a complete stranger.

You can help your loved one plan for their current and future medical and financial needs by working with them to prepare six essential legal documents; HIPAA Authorization, Healthcare Power of Attorney (POA), Living Will/Advance Healthcare Directive, Financial POA, Trust, and Will.

**See Chapter 7, "Making a Plan", for detailed information about these six must-have legal documents.

2. Be prepared for an emergency

In the event of an emergency, there are a few things you can have ready ahead of time to save yourself from panic:

- Keep a record of your loved one's doctor's office hours, including separate walk-in hours if applicable.
- Write down the location and phone numbers of the closest and highest-rated emergency rooms and urgent care clinics.
- Have a list of your loved one's allergies, medications, conditions, and blood type handy.
- Keep copies of health insurance cards and/or policy information.
- Make copies of legal medical documents (HIPAA, Healthcare POA, Living Will/Advance Healthcare Directive).
- Keep a record of your loved one's surgeries and tests (including dates and hospital locations).

3. Make a financial plan

Caring for a family member can make a serious dent in your finances. Surveys have found that over 60 percent of family caregivers say the cost of caring for an elderly loved one has impacted their ability to plan for their own financial future.

Even with the help of government-funded programs, caregivers often spend tens of thousands of dollars out of their own pockets to cover the medical costs of caring for their loved ones in their last five years of life.

For this reason, it's so important that you take steps to secure your personal finances as soon as you possibly can, and keep your own future long-term-care needs in mind.

Here are a few ways to manage your money while caregiving:

- Maximize your employer benefit programs (for working caregivers)
- Consider purchasing long-term-care insurance
- Make sure you have the right life, property, and casualty insurance
- Designate your own financial and healthcare POA
- Set up your personal will and trust

4. Reach out for help

Caregiving is hard work and you should never underestimate how mentally and emotionally exhausting it can be.

Getting help is not just a good idea, but essential if you expect to maintain your role as a caregiver for any length of time. Help can come from many people, including friends, family, neighbors, and respite workers from local organizations.

CHAPTER 5
The Physical Side of Caregiving

It's not how much you do, but how much love you put in the doing.
~ Mother Teresa

About one in ten caregivers reports that caregiving has caused their physical health to worsen.

This statistic isn't meant to scare you away from caregiving, but to make you aware of the possible negative impact caregiving can have on your health, especially if you don't learn proper stress management and other coping techniques.

Caregiving has been found to have all the features of a chronic stress experience. In other words, it creates physical and psychological strain over extended periods of time, is often uncontrollable and unpredictable, often creates secondary stress in other areas of your life (such as your work or relationships), and often requires you to be on high alert.

Not all stress is bad for you, but long-term stress of any kind is, and it can lead to serious health problems.

Some of the ways the stress of caregiving can affect your physical health include:

Weak immune system

Stress can weaken your immune system; caregivers who aren't able to keep their stress levels in check get more colds and are sick more often than non-caregivers.

Higher risk for chronic diseases

High levels of stress, especially when combined with depression, can raise your risk of health problems such as heart disease, cancer, arthritis, and diabetes.

Obesity

Stress causes weight gain in both women and men, but more so in women. Obesity increases your risk of developing other health problems such as heart disease, stroke, and diabetes.

Depression and anxiety

Caregivers, especially those who are women, are susceptible to depression and anxiety. This increases their risk of developing other health problems, such as heart disease and stroke.

Those are just a few of the ways that caregiver stress can affect your physical health. You can read more about the effects of stress in Chapter 11, "How to Manage Caregiver Stress and Prevent Burnout".

If you are experiencing any of the symptoms listed above, talk to your doctor. It's important that you get the help you need to reduce caregiver stress and help prevent any major health problems.

CHAPTER 6
The Costs of Caregiving

We make a living by what we get, but we make a life by what we give.
~ Sir Winston Churchill

Let me start by saying that this chapter isn't here to scare you away from caregiving. It's simply meant to make you aware of certain caregiving costs you may not have considered so that you can make better decisions and plans for you and your loved one. People who become full-time caregivers often look back and wish they had taken the time to better understand the financial position they would be getting themselves into.

One of the biggest hidden costs of caregiving is TIME. Most people underestimate how much time they will spend providing care. They picture themselves caring for a few hours a week for a couple of months, but end up providing care a few hours a day for a couple (or more) years.

By devoting more and more time to their loved ones, caregivers may lose more than just time. Remember, it's important that you weigh the various costs of caregiving so you will know you are making the best decisions for yourself and your loved ones.

Some additional costs of caregiving to consider include:

Lost wages

Caregivers often have to leave their jobs, reduce their hours, or take an early retirement. Leaving the workforce for a couple of months might be feasible, but doing so for a couple of years could really put you in a tough spot financially.

A recent study by MetLife found that the average caregiver's lost wages are $143,000.

Decreased employability

For those who leave the workforce to become caregivers, returning can be a challenge. Many caregivers find it very difficult to get another job after having been away for many months or years.

Lost savings and retirement

The out-of-pocket expenses of caregiving can really add up. Surveys have found that close to 50 percent of working caregivers use all or most of their savings and retirement funds. This figure is even higher for those who have left the workforce entirely.

Increased health care costs

Studies have found that least one in 10 caregivers say their role has caused their own mental and physical health to decline. Researchers have also found that caregivers have worse physical and emotional health than do non-caregivers. This equates to increased healthcare costs for caregivers, especially those who have lost their own health insurance as a result of having left their jobs to become caregivers.

The hard costs of caregiving

If you think that the previously mentioned "hidden" costs of caregiving are too high, you may want to consider alternatives to being a full-time caregiver.

Though costs may at first appear to be higher, there are a range of options that can provide the care your loved one needs without costing you time, lost wages, etc.

The following are the US national average annual costs and daily rates paid for various types of adult care:

Nursing home: semi-private room = $222/day, $81,030/year
Nursing home: private room = $248/day, $90,520/year
Assisted living = $3,550/month, $42,600/year
Home care: home health aide = $21/hour, $21,840/year
Home care: homemaker = $20/hour, $20,800/year
Adult day services = $70/day, $18,200/year

*Source: MetLife 2012 Market Survey of Long-Term Care Costs

CHAPTER 7
Making a Plan

If you fail to plan, you're planning to fail.
~ Benjamin Franklin

Most people go into caregiving without giving it much thought. They see their loved one in need, so they help. Rarely do they stop and think that their caregiving job could go on for years or that maybe they should plan things out.

If you want to be an effective caregiver, especially for someone with a chronic disease like Parkinson's, you need to know how to plan ahead. This will enable you to adapt to unexpected changes in your loved one's health and care needs.

Without the right legal and financial documentation, you and your loved one could face a whole pile of problems in an emergency. For example, doctors may refuse to discuss important medical information with you, and your loved one may not get the end-of-life care they desire. Also, it's possible that your loved one's bank accounts and property could be given to a complete stranger if your loved one becomes incapacitated.

You can help your loved one plan for their current and future medical and financial needs by working with them to prepare six legal documents:

Medical documents

HIPAA Authorization
Healthcare POA
Living Will or Advance Healthcare Directive

Financial documents

Financial POA
Trust
Will

If getting all these documents together makes you feel overwhelmed, don't worry! An elder law attorney can help prepare them for you and guide you through the process.

From someone who's been there, the work of getting these documents prepared is totally worth the peace of mind you'll have knowing that you're carrying out your loved one's wishes.

You may also want to take this time to think about your own long-term care needs and designate your own financial and healthcare POA as well as set up your personal will and trust.

Here are all those necessary legal documents explained in detail:

HIPAA Authorization (US only)

The Health Information Portability and Accountability Act (HIPAA) was created in 1996 by the US Congress to protect the privacy of your health information. This law prevents doctors and other medical professionals from discussing your health information with anyone but you unless you have provided them with a HIPAA release form. Even caregivers can't access a loved one's medical records or talk to their doctor until they sign a HIPAA form. You can get a copy of this document at your doctor's office.

Healthcare Power of Attorney (POA)

This document allows a person to grant legal authority to a trusted relative (i.e., the family caregiver) or friend to make health care decisions on their behalf. A person with a healthcare POA can determine things like where the elder lives, what they eat, who bathes them, and what medical care they receive.

NOTE: There can be some confusion when it comes to the difference between "durable" and "nondurable" powers of attorney. A durable power of attorney is a document that stays in effect indefinitely – either until you die or until you recover sufficiently to regain control over your own affairs. This is opposed to a nondurable power of attorney, which terminates when you become incapacitated or on a fixed date specified in the document.

Living Will or Advance Healthcare Directive

Living Will

This document, also known in some places as a health care declaration, lets you state what type of medical treatment you do or do not wish to receive if you are no longer able to make decisions for yourself because of illness or incapacity. Basically, it is a document that speaks for you when you're not able to do so.

A living will outlines how you want your end-of-life care to be managed (i.e., aggressive medical care versus hospice care), and may also include a Do Not Resuscitate (DNR) order or an instruction to not insert a feeding tube if you become incapable of eating on your own.

Advance Healthcare Directive

This term usually refers to a single legal document that combines a living will/healthcare declaration and a durable healthcare POA. It is currently used in most states in the US.

Technically, however, both living wills and durable POA's for health care are types of advance health care directives

The advance directive provides you with many more options, including the naming of a health care agent. With the advance directive, you can also make decisions about life-sustaining procedures in the event of a terminal condition, persistent vegetative state, AND end-stage condition. If you decide to make decisions about life-sustaining procedures in Part B of the advance directive, you should NOT fill out the living will too.

If your loved one has prepared an advance directive or living will, you should review it from time to time and update their directions if their wishes relating to health care have changed. Another reason to review this document is if there are new medical treatments available that may impact their health care decisions.

Financial Power of Attorney (POA)

A financial POA gives a trusted agent (i.e., the family caregiver or friend) the authority to act on behalf of the principal (i.e., the care-receiver) to make legally binding decisions in their financial matters. An individual with financial POA has the authority to manage a person's finances, which may include paying bills, liquidating assets to cover expenses, and making other investment decisions.

If a person doesn't have the energy, desire, or ability to deal with financial matters, this document would allow someone else to do it for him/her.

It's important to note that by granting a financial POA, principals don't give up their own power over their financial affairs; they simply delegate a representative who can sign documents, write checks, or sell real estate for them.

Trust

A trust is a legal document that lets you put conditions on how certain assets will be distributed when you die. Trusts can also help minimize gift and estate taxes.

The main difference between a trust and a will is that a trust takes effect as soon as you create it, whereas a will goes into effect only after you die.

Another difference between a trust and a will is that a will passes through probate. That means a court oversees the administration of the will and ensures the will is valid and the property gets distributed the way the deceased wanted. A trust passes outside of probate, so a court does not need to oversee the process, which can save time and money. Also, unlike a will, which becomes part of the public record, a trust can remain private.

A trust does not replace a will. Most trusts deal only with specific assets, such as life insurance or a piece of property, while a will governs distribution of nearly everything else in your estate.

Will

A will is a legal document that directs who will receive your assets and property after you die. It also appoints a legal representative to carry out your wishes.

Wills and trusts each have their advantages and disadvantages. For example, a will allows you to specify funeral arrangements and name a guardian for children, while a trust does not.

On the other hand, a trust can be used to plan for disability or to provide savings on taxes. Your elder law attorney can tell you how best to use a will and a trust in your estate plan.

~

"A living will and discussion early on in the process really helped us to make decisions that would have been impossible later on as she wasn't able to answer for herself. It helped us to let her pass with no regrets, no trips to the hospital just because, and no rest home. And most importantly, we, her children, knew exactly what she would want. Hospice was a Godsend and with the living will there was no question we were doing the things that my mother wanted." ~ Parkinson's Caregiver

CHAPTER 8
Setting Boundaries

Out of difficulties grow miracles.
~ Jean De La Breyere

Do you find yourself saying "yes" to just about everything your loved one asks you to do? Do you feel guilty for saying no? It's not uncommon for caregivers to have challenges setting limits with the loved one for whom they are caring. In fact, many say "yes" before thinking about what might be involved or what they might be committing to.

There are many possible reasons we caregivers do this: we love our spouse or parent so much and don't want to disappoint them; we love being needed; we are a helper-type person and like to fix problems; we feel responsible for the happiness of our loved one; we feel guilty if we say "no"; we don't want to be seen as neglectful; or we think we're Superwoman and should be able to do everything.

Though all these are valiant reasons for not setting limits, if you want to make it all the way in this caregiving journey, it is essential that you carefully examine your life and set clear boundaries.

In setting these boundaries, you may have to put limits on your time, money, space, or strength. Doing this will make you a stronger caregiver, one who is able to recover from or adjust easily to hardships or change.

Having boundaries that work for everyone can help caregivers continue to care while showing love and concern without the negative results of desperation, rescuing, enabling, fixing, or controlling.

Try these strategies to help set boundaries:

Evaluate

Early in your caregiving journey, have an honest, realistic talk with yourself. Think about how much of a commitment you are willing and able to make, and what you can and will do. Remember, caregiving is a team effort with your loved one. Once you have things clear in your own mind, have a family meeting to let them know what your boundaries are before problems arise.

Prioritize

Try to remember that caregiving is just ONE component of your life. Decide what matters most in your life and how you want to live out the rest of it. Do you want to maintain your career? How do you envision your marriage five or 10 years from now? Those who learn how to manage their own personal lives end up being the best caregivers.

Know their limits

Evaluate your loved one's limitations in relation to other available resources (friends, neighbors, paid help, etc.). Even though you may not always accept all your loved one's requests, let them know that you care about them.

As much as you can, try to help your loved one maintain their independence, as this will keep them happier and healthier longer.

Accept your limitations

We want to provide for all of our loved one's needs, but it's almost impossible to do so. Stick to helping only in areas that you can manage in a positive manner. Giving help grudgingly will only leave you both angry and frustrated.

Stick to your decisions

If your loved one asks you to do something that you consider unreasonable or simply more than you can manage, explain your position and make alternative suggestions.

Some people have trouble accepting the losses that can accompany Parkinson's, but as tough as it sometimes may be, you need to remember that you're not responsible for your loved one's happiness.

Detach

Initially you might think this word sounds cold and unloving, but it's really not. Detaching simply means living a life that isn't centered on someone else's. It is the ability to be close to your loved one without giving up your independence.

To be detached is to recognize your loved one's anger or frustration without taking it personally in terms of something you did or didn't do. It's avoiding jumping in right away to fix a complaint, and instead expressing interest and asking them to offer solutions.

You can detach by making caregiving a smaller part of your life. Focus on personal activities like hobbies, children, grandchildren, volunteering, getting active, learning new things, or friends.

Give yourself a break

What motivates you to be a caregiver? Think about why you took on the role. Decide to make it something you chose, not something that was forced on you.

Stay connected to your friends and family, and to the things that make you happy. Laugh and cry often, and be gentle judging yourself. Most of all, try not to take yourself too seriously!

~

"If caregivers have no boundaries and just blindly do whatever is asked of them at all times, they may burn out before they know what's happening." ~Parkinson's Caregiver

CHAPTER 9
Getting Help

I was never crippled until I lost hope.
~ Nick Vujicic

Of all the things you'll learn in your caregiving journey, this should be the first: GET HELP!

As mentioned previously, if you decide to accept the responsibilities of a caregiver, you can't - and shouldn't - try to tackle everything on your own.

As soon as possible, find all the support and respite resources that are available to you. This will save you time and effort down the road and can prove to be a lifesaver.

Here are just a few of the places and people to which family caregivers can turn for help:

- Family
- Friends
- Neighbors
- Local support groups
- Online forums
- Local home care organizations
- Local and national Parkinson's associations
- Local and national Alzheimer's associations
- Local and national administrations on aging

You can read more about how and where to get help in chapters 41-44 of this book.

--- ~ ---

PART 3
THE EMOTIONAL SIDE
OF CAREGIVING

--- ~ ---

CHAPTER 10
What to Do When You Feel Overwhelmed

I can't change the direction of the wind, but I can adjust my sails to always reach my destination.
~ Jimmy Dean

If you're feeling overwhelmed with caregiving, you're not alone. It's common to feel over your head in terms of managing the stress, worries, new skills, and piles of details involved in caring for another person.

I have personally felt this emotion several times during my caregiving journey with my mom, and each time I did, I'd like to think I got a bit better at handling it.

The reality is, there's a learning curve you have to climb in caregiving. When you start, you might imagine that every other caregiver out there has got it all together, but that's simply not true. Everyone struggles with different aspects of caregiving and has moments when they feel their life is falling apart. It's learning how to get through these struggles that makes your journey more manageable and even rewarding.

Here are a few things you can do when you find yourself feeling overwhelmed:

- Don't look at everything all at once. Remember the mantra, "one day (or hour) at a time." Break your tasks into daily and weekly chunks and try not to look too much further than a month down the road. Don't make your to-do lists too long or arduous; you'll feel like you're accomplishing more by crossing multiple things off your list.
- Put together a team. Figure out who can help, whom you can trust, and whom you are comfortable asking for what you need. If you

can spread the burdens of decision-making, hands-on care, household maintenance, and so on, it's less on you. Don't be shy about reaching out.

- Don't aim for perfection. Remember that you're not Superwoman (or man) and that you shouldn't try to be. If you always aim for the impossible, you'll always feel like you've failed. Instead, aim to do a pretty darn good job and you'll have better success reaching your goal.

- Know that you will mess up from time to time, and forgive yourself when you do. Remember: each day is a new start!

- Find out ways to be prepared for the biggest issues related to your loved one's Parkinson's so you can be ready for them.

CHAPTER 11
How to Manage Caregiver Stress and Prevent Burnout

The life of inner peace, being harmonious and without stress, is the easiest type of existence.
~ Norman Vincent Peale

It seems everyone has something to be stressed about these days. Stress is becoming so common in people's lives that you may not feel normal if you aren't stressing about something.

As a caregiver, many of the feelings you'll feel are normal, but caregiver stress can be a real problem, and if it's not managed, can lead to burnout. In addition, if that weren't enough reason to take care of your stress levels, a study from the University of California found that caregivers experiencing extreme stress have been shown to age prematurely. This level of stress can take as much as 10 years off a caregiver's life!

Stress is not just an issue for you as a caregiver, but also for your loved one with Parkinson's. It's true; stress can have a very negative impact on the symptoms of Parkinson's disease, especially tremor and mobility.

This makes it even more important for you to learn ways of controlling and managing your stress levels, as your actions affect not only your health, but that of your loved one as well.

It's a very real scenario; you get stressed out from your caregiving duties, which then makes your loved one stressed out, causing them to lose mobility, which leads to both of you being more stressed out, and so on.

If you're unsure whether you have caregiver stress, here are some common symptoms to look for:

- Depression

- Withdrawal
- Anxiety
- Insomnia
- Anger
- Exhaustion
- Headaches
- Perspiration
- Chest pain
- Hair loss
- Trouble concentrating
- Nervous habits like chain smoking
- Increased use of alcohol or stimulants
- Changes in appetite
- Back, shoulder or neck pain, muscle tension
- Weight fluctuation (gain or loss)
- High blood pressure, irregular heartbeat, palpitations
- Skin disorders (hives, eczema, psoriasis, tics, itching)
- Periodontal disease, jaw pain
- Reproductive problems/infertility
- Sexual dysfunction/lack of libido
- Weakened immune system: getting more colds, flu, infections
- Stomach/digestive problems (upset or acid stomach, cramps, heartburn, gas, irritable bowel syndrome, constipation, diarrhea)

As mentioned previously, if caregiver stress is not managed, it can lead to burnout. Hopefully, your stress levels will never get to the point of burnout, but if they do, it's important that you be able to identify whether you're in that state so you can get the help you need.

So, how do you know if you're "burned out"? If you've reached this state, you will be physically, mentally, and emotionally exhausted. Many caregivers also feel guilty if they spend time on themselves rather than on their loved one.

Burnout can happen for a number of reasons, mostly from not getting the help you need or from trying to do more than you are physically or financially able to.

The signs of caregiver burnout include all those of caregiver stress, but are more extreme. Burnout symptoms also include:

- Feeling helpless or hopeless
- Feeling constantly exhausted
- Feeling increasingly resentful
- Inability to relax
- Being on the verge of tears or crying a lot
- Overreacting to minor inconveniences
- Being short-tempered with your loved one frequently
- Losing interest in – and/or a decrease in – productivity of work
- Increasing use of medications for sleeplessness, anxiety, depression
- A change in attitude - positive and caring to negative and unconcerned
- Increasing thoughts of death

The following strategies can help you manage stress and prevent burnout. Please note that not all techniques work for everyone, so you may have to experiment a little to find something that works for you. Remember that the key to successful stress management is practice.

Prioritize your to-do list

If you're like most caregivers, your to-do lists can get pretty long and cumbersome. Accept that you can't always get everything done in one day. Prioritize your lists, set up a daily routine and break large tasks into small do-able chunks to help you get more things done.

Say "no"

Say "no" to social requests that are draining or stressful (i.e., hosting holiday get-togethers). Knowing your limits and what you can handle is important so you can make sure not to over extend yourself.

Deep breathing

Take slow, deep breaths from your diaphragm. Breathe in through your nose and out through your mouth. Count to five as you breathe in and five as you breathe out. Do this several times until you begin to feel more relaxed.

Progressive relaxation

Get in a comfortable position, close your eyes, and slowly focus on relaxing different parts of your body, one at a time. Start at your head and work down to your feet. There are many different relaxation CD's or MP3's out there that can guide you.

Relax with music

There are many benefits of music, including relaxation and pain management. You can find all kinds of relaxation materials in bookstores and music stores or over the Internet. You may have to experiment a little to find something that works for you.

Music is good not only for you, but also for the person for whom you are caring, making it easier to work with them.

We use music as much as possible to get Mom going when she's "stuck" somewhere, as well as to lift her mood when she's in a funk.

Whether we have her hooked up to an iPod, have her favorite music playing on a stereo or are simply humming a marching tune loudly along beside her, it's incredible to watch how she can go from being completely immobile to practically running across the room!

Meditate or pray

Did you know that both meditation and prayer have scientifically proven health benefits? When you meditate or pray, the activity of your brain moves from the right frontal cortex (where stress lives) to the calm left frontal cortex.

This results in feeling relaxed, which then slows down your breathing. When your breathing slows to six breaths a minute, your breath becomes aligned with the rhythms in your heart, which is good for your cardiovascular health.

Other physical benefits of meditation and prayer include anti-aging, decreased blood pressure, higher skin resistance, deep rest, and easier breathing.

Some mental benefits include greater creativity, decreased anxiety and depression, improved learning and memory, and increased happiness and emotional stability.

Pamper yourself

Set aside time to treat yourself to something you wouldn't normally do. Give yourself a manicure and pedicure, soak in a hot bubble bath, get a massage, engage in some retail therapy (shopping!), or have a movie marathon with all your favorites.

Attend a support group

Even though it seems that you have no time for your support group now, it is more important than ever to attend. Some people attend more than one group.

Participants in your support group will understand how much the inability of some family members and friends to be with you and your care-receiver now hurts, how hard it is to remain patient with some of your care-receiver's behaviors, and how frustrating it can be to "navigate the system" to get affordable assistance.

Keep in touch

Find a friend or family member whom you trust to talk to and share your feelings and frustrations with.

Try counseling

Unfortunately, many caregivers don't take time for counseling until their caregiving gig is over, but it's a good idea to talk with a counselor while in the midst of caregiving.

Consider professional counseling to deal with difficult emotions, including anger, anxiety, grief, and guilt. This may be especially important if you're caring for someone who has both Parkinson's and dementia, as that can be extra trying on you.

A counselor can help you see things clearly and set goals for maintaining your own life while caregiving.

Get regular check-ups

Visit your doctor regularly to get your health checked. Whether it be a mammogram, prostrate test, colon cancer test, or a flu or pneumonia shot, it's important that you schedule time for whatever tests you may need. Think of it as preventative maintenance for your caregiving machine. After all, if your health declines, you won't be able to care for your loved one.

If you and your doctor agree that you need to take medications because of stress, consider adding them to help in addition to the other strategies mentioned here.

Exercise

It is a well-known fact that exercise is not only good for your physical health, but also a great way to reduce stress and anxiety and relieve depression.

Exercise is important for both the caregiver and the person with PD. If it works for both of you, you may choose to attend an exercise, yoga, or Tai Chi class together at a local community or fitness center.

Other exercises you may want to choose are walking (outside or on a treadmill), swimming, dancing, or lifting weights (appropriate for your level of fitness).

Whatever you choose, make sure it's something you like to do and just keep moving!

Laugh a little

Try to maintain a sense of humor while caregiving. This may sound very simple, but one of the biggest ways you can reduce stress is through laughter.

Yes, laughter really can be the best medicine. Recent studies suggest that laughter can help in many ways to heal the mind and body.

There are even "laughter clubs" that are emerging across the US, Canada, and even the world that are designed to get people laughing.

If you think this sounds crazy or that it couldn't work, check out their website at: www.worldlaughtertour.com.

Try pet therapy

If you have a pet, you probably don't need convincing that animals can have a positive effect on your mood and overall health. Holding or playing with your dog or cat can provide much-needed comfort and laughs.

If you don't have a pet, try spending time with one. Even something as simple as watching the fish in an aquarium or a goldfish pond can be very relaxing.

Get help!

Don't forget to ask for help from family, friends, support groups, and your local Parkinson's foundation. Tell them if you're feeling burnt out by caregiver stress. You'll be surprised at who comes out of the woodwork when you let people know you need help.

CHAPTER 12
Keeping Your Cool:
How to Stay Patient During Those Trying Times

In all things it is better to hope than to despair.
~ Johann Wolfgang von Goethe

Anger isn't an emotion I'm overly comfortable with; I usually try to avoid it if I can. Sure, if you push my buttons over and over or offend my deepest convictions I will stand up for myself, but in general I try to steer clear of most situations if and when they get volatile.

When it comes to caregiving, I have to admit I've had a least a few moments when I've lost my patience and not been as cool as I'd like to have been with my mom.

Here's some comforting news: all caregivers "lose it" sometimes. We lose patience, we yell, we have meltdowns. The important thing is what we do with that anger.

There are several things you can do to help manage this difficult emotion:

- Remind yourself that you're angry and frustrated with the situation, NOT your loved one.
- Don't beat yourself up about it – forgive yourself and move on.
- Acknowledge that you're exhausted and emotional and know that it's common for caregivers to snap at their loved ones once in a while, especially when you're in this state.
- Take deep, slow breaths to get control over your body – then you'll have a better chance of gaining control of your emotions. This sounds simple, but it works!

- As always, reach out for help! Getting help to ease your caregiver load can give you much-needed rest and help prevent potential anger episodes.
- Find ways to let off steam – exercise, write in a journal, go out with a friend, or just plain ol' scream (somewhere private, of course)!
- If you find yourself getting angry frequently, talk to a counselor, therapist, or clergyperson to help you find ways to manage that.

CHAPTER 13
How to Deal with Guilt

When you exhaust all possibilities remember this - you haven't.
~ Thomas Edison

I wish someone had taught me early on in my caregiving journey about guilt. I wrestled with this emotion for a very long time, not knowing what to do with it or how common it was.

Here's a news flash about caregiving: you're going to feel guilty a lot of the time. Guilty for not doing enough. Guilty for not being there enough. Guilty for losing your temper, making wrong decisions, or breaking promises.

Guilt was such a part of my life that I felt guilty every time I was having fun and she wasn't. That feeling still creeps up from time to time when I'm out enjoying myself.

Here are some key points and strategies to deal with guilt:

- Remind yourself that guilt is NORMAL.
- Acknowledge that you're doing your best.
- Realize that no matter how much time you spend with your loved one trying to meet all their needs, guilt will make you feel like it's never enough. Guilt can eat you alive – don't let it.
- Try a mantra ("I love my mom, I'm doing the best I can.").
- Don't fall into the "I shoulda or coulda" trap – things are what they are and stewing about it just wastes time and energy.
- Know that there are two types of guilt: good guilt and bad guilt. Good guilt can help you make positive changes by pointing out little things to improve in your behavior. For example, if you feel guilty because you were impatient with your loved one, good guilt will remind you to try to be a bit more patient next time. Bad guilt,

45

on the other hand, does nothing for us except make us feel guilty about a situation we can't control or one that is actually good for us (e.g., hiring home care because you can't do it all yourself).

- Instead of focusing on the things you're not doing right for your loved one, focus on the things you are doing right.

CHAPTER 14
How to Cope with Loneliness

Remember we're all in this alone.
~ Lily Tomin

Caregiving can be a lonely job. It can isolate you from friends because they can't relate to your demanding life. It can make you feel so tired or depressed that going out with them feels like too much work, so instead you stay at home, feeling lonely.

If you're experiencing feelings of loneliness, know that many other caregivers out there are feeling the same. With just a bit of effort, you can help lessen this feeling by keeping connected with the right friends and/or family members.

Though some friendships may fade, your close friends will stand by you if you can "help them help you." Here are some ways you can do this:

- Understand your friends' limits – not everyone will be able or willing to take the long caregiver journey with you – it's tough.
- Give direction – sometimes friends want to help but don't know how. They may also find it hard to relate to you now. If this is the case, talk to them and let them know what you need; that sometimes all you want is for them to be there and listen.
- Hang on to your friends and let them know how much you appreciate them.
- Get out once in a while! Though you may not feel like socializing, just being around others can keep depression at bay. Go to the movies, go out for lunch, or go on a walk with one or more friends. Force yourself to take a break from caregiving at least once a week!

CHAPTER 15
How to Handle Depression

Some days there won't be a song in your heart. Sing anyway.
~ Emory Austin

While I was battling depression in my teens, I remember my mom telling me that she couldn't be happy until I was better. "A mother is only as happy as her most unhappiest child," she'd say. In caring for my mom, I've come to understand what she meant back then.

Caring for someone with Parkinson's definitely has its share of challenges. One of the biggest is dealing with the depression that can accompany it. If you're not diligent, your loved one's depression can cause you to get depressed as well, so learning about this side of Parkinson's is very important for both of you.

Depression is very common in people with Parkinson's and can happen as a result of the disease and/or because of the side effects of the drugs taken for it. If your loved one suffers from depression, it will most definitely affect you, too.

Because depression is the number-one issue that prevents people from having a happy and full life, it is extremely important that you be on the lookout for signs of depression in your loved one.

Depression can also increase the physical effects of Parkinson's disease and may cause a progression of the disease.

If you observe your loved one experiencing five or more of the following symptoms for longer than two weeks at a time, you should contact their doctor:

- Depressed mood
- An inability to find pleasure in things that were once pleasurable
- Sleep disturbances (inability to sleep or sleeping excessively)

- Change in appetite
- Fatigue
- Altered level of activity
- Difficulty with concentration
- Low self-esteem
- Thoughts of death

The good news is that for most people with Parkinson's disease, depression can be controlled. Depression may be treated with psychological therapy, as well as with medications. People seem to do better when they receive both psychological and drug treatments.

Psychological therapy can help people with Parkinson's regain their sense of self-worth even though they may not be able to do as much anymore. It can also help the person maintain good relationships with caregivers and family members despite having to depend on them more.

There are many anti-depressant medications available, each with its own advantages and disadvantages. Most people with Parkinson's disease should not take Ascendin (amoxipine) because this medication could temporarily worsen Parkinson's disease symptoms. Your loved one's doctor will know which ones are best for them.

*Note: Make sure you check with your pharmacist about taking any new medications (like antidepressants), as there may be some that are not compatible with your loved one's PD medications.

~

Here's a little story to finish this topic of depression. You may wish to share this with your loved one if they need a little encouragement.

When my mom was first diagnosed, a family member suggested she go to a support group for people with Parkinson's. When she arrived, she encountered a room full of sad-looking people in wheelchairs. This was very discouraging and depressing for her, as she barely had any noticeable symptoms of PD at this point.

Now, in that moment she made a crucial decision. She decided that as much as possible, she wasn't going to let Parkinson's bring her down.

She also decided that she was going to do all she could to keep her independence for as long as possible.

"Don't let anyone take away your independence," Mom used to say. In other words, don't give up and say, "Oh well, I have Parkinson's. I guess I'm doomed to X, Y, or Z."

Mom made it over 15 years with Parkinson's before she relied on a wheelchair for any length of time. Now, we all know that every case of Parkinson's is different and maybe my mom got "the good kind," but I believe that it has also been her strong will, determination, faith, and positive outlook that have helped her live for 25 years with this disease.

CHAPTER 16
How to Cope with
Worry of the Unknown

Worry often gives a small thing a big shadow.
~ Swedish Proverb

I always thought my mom to be a bit of a worrywart, which is probably where I got my worrying tendencies. It's not like I don't know it's bad for me – I *know* it is – but facing giants like Parkinson's and dementia has made me more worried about the future than ever before.

Intellectually I know that no one can predict or control the future, but it's hard for me to not wonder if I will suffer the same fate as my mom.

If there's one thing in life I used to think was controllable, it was one's health. Just eat right, exercise regularly, and avoid stress and you'll make it 'til at least your 70s with no major health issues. But when Mom was diagnosed with Parkinson's in her late 40s and my sister with cancer in her mid-40s, I had to face the fact that maybe we can't entirely control our health.

Over the past year I've been working on eliminating my fears of future ill health and other unknowns. I now know that fear of the unknown is nothing more than a mental obstacle. This obstacle has been getting in the way of my being able to live my life to the fullest, but at least now that I'm aware of that fact, I am doing something about it.

If you've been burdened with fear and worry of the unknown, you'll be happy to know that you can get rid of these by applying some of the following techniques in your life:

Understand your fear

To best fight your fear, you need to understand the cause of it. Fear is a natural human instinct and almost all of us fear something in our lives.

Fear of the unknown stems from certain things, situations, or memories in life.

Ask yourself, "What do I fear the most? What situations do I frequently avoid in my day-to-day life?" Once you are able to figure out the root cause of the fear, you will find it easier to combat it.

Educate yourself

In some cases, fear of the unknown can be based on certain factors that are beyond our control. In these cases, educating yourself about the fear and learning about the actual risk is the best way to ease your fear.

For instance, if you fear being diagnosed with Parkinson's down the road, leaning about the stats of who gets PD and what the risk factors are may help you.

I sometimes go down the road of, "If I get Parkinson's, who will take care of me? How will I pay for all my medical costs? Will I end up with dementia in the end?" These are all legit questions, and the first two I can somewhat plan for if I choose to, which helps ease my fear. I can't control whether or not I get dementia, though, so worrying about that is just wasted time and energy.

Mom used to fear that she'd get trapped in the house in a fire or tornado when she was immobile and nobody would be there to help her out. This fear may appear dramatic, but I understood the helplessness she felt when her PD made her stuck in place, so I assured her over and over again that someone would be there to help her in an emergency.

Our minds tend to think about the worst-case scenarios, but the worst may not happen at all. Michael J. Fox once said, "If you imagine the worst-case scenario, and it comes true, you've lived it twice." I try to remind myself that worrying doesn't do anything other than make me more stressed and susceptible to illness.

Confront your fear!

Often our tendency is to run from situations that induce fear; in the process, we may lose certain opportunities in life. If you want to experience all that life has to offer, you must move out of your comfort zone and confront your fears!

Visualize and meditate

Other ways to fight fear of the unknown are visualization and meditation. These techniques will help you focus on the positives rather than on your fear.

To do this, find a quiet place away from any noise so that you can meditate peacefully. Once in your quiet place, stay seated and visualize in your mind how you are going to fight your fear step by step. Imagine yourself conquering your fears every day. Winning the battle in your mind will help you take real action.

Take baby steps

If you're living with a fear that can cause no real harm to you, take baby steps to eliminate it. For instance, if you have a fear of public speaking, speak in front of a small group of friends or family. Taking baby steps will go a long way in helping you fight your fear over a period of time.

Fight fear with fun!

Don't take your life too seriously. Once time is gone, you can't get it back. Wasting too much time being worried or fearful of the unknown is just that – a waste.

Humor is another great way to get rid of the fear of the unknown. The idea is to ease your mind to ensure that there are no unwanted thoughts troubling you. Hang around with your friends and spend time watching funny movies.

~

"We try not to be naïve, keep informed with all the latest information, laugh A LOT, while planning realistically for what might be. It's a fine balance."
~ Parkinson's Caregiver

CHAPTER 17
How to Deal with Resentment

The greatest act of faith some days is
to simply get up and face another day.
~ Amy Gatliff

"I am sitting here trying to understand how to deal with the loneliness and resentment I feel for giving up my own home and life. I have been sleeping on the floor at my parents' for the last two years and have given up all but my job to care for them. Don't get me wrong, I love my parents to death but I have been caring for my dad (who has Parkinson's) for about 10 years now. It started out slowly but now is a full-time job."
– Parkinson's Caregiver

This sentiment, shared with me by a fellow Parkinson's caregiver, is one felt by many caregivers. Whether it be directed towards Parkinson's, the situation in general, or your loved one, it's tough for even the most willing caregivers to fend off resentment all of the time.

Resentment is a very human emotion, so don't beat yourself up if you feel it towards the person you're caring for. Almost all caregivers feel this way at one time or another. After all, it's hard accepting that the life you planned and hoped to have with your loved one isn't going to come to fruition.

Here are a few things to help you deal with resentment:

- Remind yourself that, above all, it's the situation you're resentful of. It's rarely the person in your care who's causing your feelings; what you're upset about is almost always the disease, the burden of caregiving, and the changes to all your lives. Try not to feel guilty for feeling this way.
- As hard as it may be at first, try to let go of some of the past and future. If you dwell on what might have been, you'll find

resentment creeping in. Instead, focus on being in the present and look for the good things in the life you share with your loved one.

- Find an outlet for resentment so that it doesn't consume you. Be it exercising, talking with a friend, writing in a journal, or even screaming it out (somewhere private), it is important that you have healthy ways to vent your feelings.

- Don't let caregiving be the only thing in your life. Make time to do things that make you happy – this will make you a better caregiver in the end.

--- ~ ---

PART 4
GETTING PRACTICAL:
GENERAL CAREGIVING ISSUES

--- ~ ---

CHAPTER 18
How to Help When Help Isn't Wanted

Life can only be understood backwards; but it must be lived forwards.
~ Soren Kierkegaard

It's tough to see your loved one go through the challenges that come with Parkinson's. Progressively losing mobility is just one of the many losses they have to deal with, and each loss brings with it a sense that your loved one is slowly losing their independence and freedom. These losses can also deal a significant blow to their self-esteem.

Many aging adults refuse help from their younger family members because it reminds them of their age. Even though family members mean well, sometimes they offer help in a way that challenges their older loved one's identity as an independent adult.

The thing is, most old people don't need or want to be reminded that they are old. In fact, studies have found that this is the main reason they refuse help. When their identities are threatened, older people may even lash out, sometimes in a dangerous manner, to prove their youth.

As a caregiver for someone with Parkinson's, you'll want to keep your loved one safe while they get the care and help they need. The challenge will be to do this without overstepping your boundaries, causing them to become resentful and resist your help.

Here are a few ways to help your loved one when they're resistant:

Ask; don't order

If your loved one believes that asking for help was their idea, they may be more likely to accept your help. If you start by lending a hand with just those things for which your loved one admits to needing help, they may be more receptive to any future suggestions you have regarding their need for outside assistance.

Often you may find the person you are caring for getting frustrated because they are unable to complete certain daily activities that they once were able to. One common area of frustration is walking. Depending on the stage of Parkinson's in which they are, you may be able to help a person with Parkinson's disease overcome some of their difficulties.

For example, Mom frequently has trouble walking when her meds start to wear off. Often when this happens, she starts to get frustrated and forgets that she knows other ways of getting from A to B.

Here's where the caregiver can jump in and offer some suggestions to help her out. In this case, we simply suggest to Mom, "Why don't you try walking sideways?" Mom does, and immediately she is on her way.

It's important that we not tell Mom what to do, but suggest or ask her if she'd like to try another method of walking. This way, Mom is still choosing what she would like to do, and doesn't feel ordered around.

R-E-S-P-E-C-T

This little word can go a long way in your caregiving journey. Remember it in everything you do with your loved one, as it is the foundation upon which all good relationships are built.

One way you can show respect to your care receiver is to ask them for permission before you rush in to help them with something. For example, before you assume that it's okay for you to sit in on their doctor's appointments, ask them how they feel about that. If they don't want you in the exam room, you can always wait outside and talk to their doctor about your concerns once the appointment is over.

Ask to help with little things first

Even if your loved one doesn't want your help with a certain task, they may allow you to help them if you ask to help out a little. Just make sure that when you do lend them a hand, you don't end up taking over. Remember, the goal is to help them keep their independence, sense of purpose, and self-worth.

If your loved one needs help with their daily activities, you may suggest a home support worker or someone who can help them out from time to time (like another family member or a friend). Sometimes people accept help from "outsiders" more readily than they do from their close family members.

Also, you could suggest that the support worker (or whomever) come out on a trial basis. That way your loved can see the benefits of having outside help.

Keep them safe

Always remember that safety should come first. If you have to assume total control of a task to make sure that your loved one is safe, that is more important than anything.

CHAPTER 19
What NOT to do When Caregiving

It is not the mountain we conquer but ourselves.
~ Edmund Hillary

Caregiving is a process of trial and error. You will make mistakes from time to time, but learning from them is the key. To help you out in your caregiving journey, there are a few things you'll want to avoid doing.

Here a few of the "don'ts" in caregiving:

Don't try to "fix" everything all at once

You've probably been told this before, but it's worth repeating; pick your battles. Your loved one may need help with many tasks and you may discover that they want things done in a way that is different from the way you'd do them. Remember that your goal should be to help them, not "fix them." Prioritize their needs and work with them to tackle one task at a time.

Don't patronize

Sometimes, as an aging loved one becomes more fragile, we start treating them more like children than adults. Don't do this. Even if you're caring for someone with dementia, be careful not to talk down to them. Treat your loved one the way you'd want to be treated.

Don't interrupt

Make sure you're really listening to what your loved one is saying. Try not to interrupt or fill the silence during a conversation. When it's your turn to speak, summarize what you think your loved one just said and then ask them if you have correctly interpreted their sentiments.

Don't give advice unless it's asked for

This is an especially important tip for adult children who are looking after aging parents. Your mother and father are used to providing you with advice and guidance. When this dynamic begins to shift, it may start to lower their self-esteem and make them feel out of control. Getting an outside expert—such as a financial advisor or an elder law attorney—to provide professional guidance can make an elder more receptive to new information.

Don't forget about how they feel

Put yourself in their shoes. Remember, your loved one is probably feeling as though they are losing control over their own life. In their mind, their freedom and independence are being threatened. Always show empathy and sensitivity towards them.

Don't be argumentative

One thing I learned very early on in my caregiving journey is that I am not my mother. She has different ways of seeing things and wanting to do things, and because of this we didn't always see eye to eye.

Remember to acknowledge your loved one's questions, concerns, and viewpoints. Compromising was something I learned to do to reduce the number of our disagreements.

Don't forget your TONE

Though your patience will be tested throughout your caregiving journey, it's important that you pay attention to your tone when you're talking with your loved one. Speak calmly and avoid raising your voice or being condescending. Doing so can quickly turn a conversation into an argument, which can then escalate into something even bigger.

Also, if your loved one has difficulty hearing, keep your voice low and make sure to enunciate your words so that they can really hear what you're saying. Nothing's worse than an argument starting over something you didn't even say!

CHAPTER 20
Long-Distance Caregiving

I never worry about action, but only about inaction.
~ Winston Churchill

Caring for my mom while living 2500 miles away has definitely been a challenge. When I lived nearby it was a lot easier to know how she was doing and what her needs were. Though I've tried my best to keep up to date with her health and to help her via telephone, sometimes it feels like it's just not enough.

I've gone through all kinds of emotions, including guilt over not being able to visit more often, frustration over not being able to help as much as I once could, and worry over the level of care she's receiving. I've struggled with letting go and depending on others to care for her.

If you're a long-distance caregiver, you can probably relate to some of what I just described. Maybe you spend your long weekends or vacations visiting your loved one, hoping and praying that each time you visit they'll still be okay.

Apparently we're not alone in this. A recent online poll for caregivers found that almost one-third of all caregivers care for their loved ones from a distance, and most struggle with the things I just mentioned.

Though there will be challenges along the way, there are some things you can do to make caring for your loved one from a distance easier:

Communicate

It may sound simple, but communication is so important in caregiving. Communicating with those who are involved with caring for your loved one locally can help you keep on top of their changing needs.

This will help you know if or when they need more skilled help in their home or, if they're in a care facility, what changes in care, medications, diet, etc., need to be made to their daily regimen.

So, what can long-distance relatives do to be helpful, short of moving back home? Let your loved one and the primary caregiver know that you are still there for them.

Get local help

If you find that you can't keep track of all that is needed for your loved one from afar, there's a relatively new service that may be able to help you. Consider hiring a geriatric care manager (also known as Aging Life Care) who can be your liaison and provide services, including arranging financial, legal, and medical services and assisting with a move from home to a care facility.

It is important to note that not all geriatric care managers are required to be certified by their state or the federal government, so make sure that you interview them yourself and/or do a thorough check with their organization before you hire them.

Be kind to yourself

Long-distance caregiving can be emotionally draining. If you're like me, you'll probably experience a range of emotions like those I mentioned earlier.

Getting a support system in place is really important to help you with all these emotions. Sometimes after a Skype call with my mom, I just need a hug. Thankfully, I have a very supportive husband who's always there to give me one (or more!).

Connect with family

If your family doesn't get together very often, you may find that when you do, your talks tend to center on the subject of Parkinson's and your loved one's care needs. Though this may be necessary, sometimes we need to be reminded to take a break from that and talk about other things. A good heart-to-heart talk with my sister is something we both benefit from.

Set up weekly phone or Skype dates

I always look forward to Mondays and Thursdays at 5 PM. That's when I get to Skype (video call) my mom to see how she's doing and tell her my swimming stories. If you ask me, video calling is one of the greatest communication inventions in recent times. It has made such a positive difference for my mom and me while I've been her long-distance caregiver.

Many parents with adult children think that they are bothering them by calling, so they don't. Another reason they don't call is because they think, as my mom used to say, "It costs a fortune." Even though she's wrong (most Skype calls are free or virtually free), I make it easier on her by being the one who picks up the phone.

Setting up a regular Skype (or phone) date with your loved one is not only a great way to see how they're doing and get a chance to share your life with them, it also gives your loved one something to look forward to regularly, which can mean a lot.

Get peace of mind

The biggest way to find peace of mind in caregiving is knowing that your loved one is safe and that their care needs are being met.

Obtaining this information and "staying in the loop" can be hard when you live far away. Often you get secondhand information about your loved one, making it hard to know exactly what's going on.

To remedy this, you want to get as many eyes on the situation as you can. Connect with those who interact with your loved one, whether it be your loved one's primary caregiver at home or nurses and support workers at a care facility where they live. If they go for a doctor's appointment, call afterwards and ask how it went.

Take the time to find professionals who can help your loved one. If need be, hire an elder law attorney to make sure your loved one's finances and insurance needs are taken care of.

Plan for the future

Planning for an emergency isn't exactly "fun," but it can be helpful. Of course, you can't plan for every possible scenario, but knowing what you might do if your loved one has a fall or if their condition worsens can help you face and deal with the situation more easily if it does happen.

I have to admit that my family didn't plan for when my mom first had a bad fall and had to be rushed to the emergency room to get 16 stitches in her head. It was scary, but thankfully my sister and I were close by and were able to be with and comfort my mom while she was in the hospital.

All of us caregivers dread getting that emergency phone call. I hate thinking about it, but I know that if it happens again, my family and I will get through it.

Educate yourself

If you're not already versed in "All things Parkinson's," you should at least have a basic understanding of the disease. This will help you support your loved one and anyone who may be caring for them close by.

You can start by Googling your National Parkinson's Foundation or going to AllAboutParkinsons.com. There you can find information on diagnosis, symptoms, treatment options, nutrition and exercise regimens, and a whole lot more.

Make sure you know your loved one's current needs and the medications they're taking. Keep a contact list of their doctor, neurologist, pharmacist, and any health care workers who are involved in caring for your loved one.

You may also want to have financial and legal documents available in case they're needed.

Check in on finances

Talking about money is always tricky, so be sure that when you do talk to your loved one about this topic, you do so tactfully.

Many people won't ask for financial help even if they're in dire straits, but if there's a need and you can help, offer to do so. If your loved one won't accept monetary assistance, they may accept your help in purchasing needed items for their care, or allow you to help pay for utility bills, transportation costs, or housecleaning or yard services.

Be kind to your loved one's caregivers

Let those who are caring for your loved one close by know that they are appreciated. Whether it be something as simple as a thank-you card, a bouquet of flowers, or something more elaborate like a gift basket, such gifts of thanks can mean a lot to someone who may be tired from all the demands of caregiving.

Visit when you can

Decide how many times a month or year you can afford to visit and budget for it. When you do visit, try to do so when your loved one has an appointment with the neurologist so that you can be there for it. This can be beneficial for both you and the doctor.

Also, when you're visiting don't add to the primary caregiver's stress level by asking or expecting them to put you up or take care of you.

Know that all visits are important

If your loved one has developed dementia along with their Parkinson's, it's likely that they don't connect with you the way they used to when you visit. Many long-distance caregivers find this very painful and wonder if their visits are still valuable.

I experienced this very recently while visiting my mom in the nursing home where she currently lives. A few times she's been so agitated that I questioned whether my being there was making her life better or worse.

That's when I reminded myself that I wasn't there just to visit. I used some of my time to talk with the nurses, personal support workers, and volunteers who are all part of Mom's care team.

This helped me get a better idea of how she was doing on a day-to-day basis and in what ways I could help her. Something as simple as finding out that she needed long socks (her precious short ones kept falling off during episodes of dyskinesia) made me feel better, as it gave me something specific that I could do to help her.

I was also able to speak to her doctor, who agreed to make a medication change (I discovered that Mom was being given unnecessary pain meds for a fall she had months ago), and was able to talk to Mom's physical therapist about making changes to her wheelchair to make it more comfortable for her.

Help the primary caregiver

Living far away may mean that you can't personally cover for your loved one's primary caregiver, but you can offer to pay for respite care. This could be at an extended care facility or at your home if your loved one is able to travel.

If and when the time comes, don't shy away from agreeing to a decision to have your loved one moved to a residential care facility. Respect the fact that you're not the one providing the day-to-day care or that you don't know how much of a burden the primary caregiver has.

Try not to let finances or egos get in the way of doing what's best for those whose lives are most affected.

Long-distance caregiving "NO's"

As a long-distance caregiver, you have ways to support your loved one's primary caregiver. The following are a few points to remember:

- Don't underestimate anything. Being away from your loved one may make you susceptible to underestimating the severity of their day-to-day symptoms and what level of caregiver burden they can be. Providing physical care, particularly for someone with advanced Parkinson's, can be physically demanding, so be sensitive to the primary caregiver's needs.

- Be careful about offering advice. As you aren't with your loved one on a day-to-day basis, you may not have an accurate reading of how things are going with them. If you have points of wisdom you'd like to offer your loved one's primary caregiver, do so carefully and avoid criticizing them.

- Don't make promises you can't keep. Though you may mean well, it's important that you don't make promises to your loved one that you may not be able to keep. Instead of saying things like "Don't worry, Mom, we'd never put you in a home," be empathetic and tell your loved one that you will talk about other options if and when the time comes.

CHAPTER 21
How Long Will My Caregiving Job Last?

Never be afraid to trust an unknown future to a known God.
~ Corrie ten Boom

One of the many questions you may be asking yourself as a caregiver is how long your job will last. This is a tough question to answer because, as you've probably already heard, Parkinson's varies from person to person, and so will caregiving jobs.

In most cases, Parkinson's disease progresses slowly and, on average, people with it live between 10 and 20 years after diagnosis. These numbers should be put into perspective with respect to how old the individual was at diagnosis.

The average length of time spent as a caregiver is about five years, but, again, that will depend on what stage your loved one was in when you took over your caregiving role.

Factors such as being diagnosed later in life, scoring poorly on movement tests, experiencing delusions, hallucinations, or other psychotic symptoms, and developing dementia have all been associated with a shorter life expectancy. In addition, men with Parkinson's are more likely to die early than are women.

The fact is, if you decide to care for your loved one through the end stages of Parkinson's (and not move them into a full-time care facility), you will most likely be facing a caregiving journey of several years.

CHAPTER 22
What to Do When No One Will Help

You have within you, right now, everything you need to deal with whatever the world can throw at you.
~ Brian Tracy

Caregiving is tough and even more so when other family members won't help and you feel that you have to do it all on your own. It's not uncommon for there to be one person in the family who has to "step up" and take on most of the burden of caregiving. If this has happened to you, you know how it can make you feel: resentful, stressed out, and overwhelmed.

So why does this happen? Everyone copes with Parkinson's in different ways. Some family members may go into denial, some may get depressed, and others may make themselves busy trying to do everything.

You may look at a family member and think that they aren't helping, but it could just be their way of dealing with a particular problem. This is why talking to your family is so important.

Many conflicts can be avoided through simple communication. This doesn't necessarily mean that your family members will help out, but at least by talking with them you can get a better understanding of where they're coming from.

Here are a few things to keep in mind when no one will help:

- Understand that everyone reacts and copes in different ways.
- Before you give up on receiving help from family members, make sure you have asked them directly for help. Sometimes caregivers complain about siblings not helping when they actually haven't given them a chance to do so.
- Make a care plan that can be changed as needed.

- Get respite care to prevent burnout! Find out what resources and services are available in the area (things like transportation, meal delivery, companionship, etc.).
- If family won't help, find alternate sources of help. Don't waste energy being angry and frustrated about it. It's not worth it.
- Keep asking for help until you get the kind and amount you need!

--- ~ ---

PART 5
GETTING PRACTICAL:
CAREGIVING FOR
PARKINSON'S

--- ~ ---

CHAPTER 23
Parkinson's Caregiving: Early Stages

To care for those who once cared for us is one of the highest honors.
~ Tia Walker

As you begin the journey of Parkinson's with your loved one, you'll probably have a lot of questions. You'll also most likely have a lot of new information and advice thrown at you that you'll have to sift through.

Because Parkinson's affects everyone differently, no caregiving journey will be exactly the same. As a caregiver for someone with Parkinson's, you have to learn and adapt as you go. Just remember that your journey will be a team effort and you don't have to – and shouldn't – go it alone!

Here are some suggestions to help you care for your loved one in the early stages of Parkinson's:

Educate yourself

When you're first starting out as a Parkinson's caregiver, you'll want to learn the basics of Parkinson's. Things like identifying the various stages, learning and managing symptoms, and understanding medications and their side effects are some of the main points you should know.

There are many resources available for caregivers, but the best place to start is your National Parkinson's Foundation. They can quickly and easily direct you to the best places for the resources you want and need. You can find them online.

Learning about Parkinson's is just one aspect of educating yourself, as you'll want to learn about the specific ways in which the disease is affecting your loved one as well. As you care for them, observe them closely to detect any changes in their motor function (ability to move) and mood.

Because your loved one might not be aware of their changing abilities, you can be their extra set of eyes. This will enable you to give them better emotional and physical support.

As mentioned earlier, caring for someone with Parkinson's is a process of learning and adapting as you go. The more you can learn about Parkinson's in the early stages, the more you will be able to take part in health care discussions and make informed decisions in the future.

Learn to adapt

When you first hear that your loved one has Parkinson's, it can come as a real shock. Your life may seem like it has been turned completely upside down, and you may feel unqualified for taking on the caregiving role.

Feeling this way is common; however, becoming a caregiver is a role you can learn and grow into.

You may have many questions, including whether or not you should get a second opinion, how you will share the diagnosis with the family, and how you will balance your needs with those of your loved one. These are all good questions to ask.

In many cases, getting a second opinion is a good idea, as long as it's from someone who's qualified – like a neurologist who specializes in Parkinson's.

When it comes to sharing the diagnosis with family and friends, talk with your loved one about how you want to do this. If you have children living at home, make sure you tell them in an age-appropriate way.

Because Parkinson's is a progressive disease, your loved one's needs will change. As they do, so will your caregiving responsibilities. Communicate with your loved one about your needs as well to make sure that you are taking care of yourself throughout your caregiving journey.

Be patient

One very important skill you'll need to learn or develop as a caregiver for someone with Parkinson's is patience.

Some days your loved one's symptoms will be very obvious, while other days not as much. Ask if you can help your loved one with tasks, but don't assume that they want help, because they may not. Be patient and allow them to do things on their own, even if it takes longer. Trying to rush your loved one will only get them frustrated and stressed and slow them down even more.

It takes time to learn everything there is to know about caring for someone with Parkinson's, so don't forget to be patient with yourself as well.

Provide reassurance

Providing your loved one with reassurance, especially in the early stages after diagnosis, can really help. Remind them that Parkinson's disease progresses slowly in most people, and that they can still live a full life.

Because depression is so common in people with Parkinson's, it never hurts to offer a hug or two, or any kind of physical touch. Let your loved one know you're in this together.

Talk to someone who's been there

It may be helpful for you and your loved one to talk to an experienced caregiver – one who has "been there, done that." He or she can share strategies on how to deal with the various situations you may face.

They may also be able to give you the reassurance that Parkinson's is a slowly progressing disease for most people and that it can be lived with – and lived with well.

Try a support group

Attending a support group can be a good way to educate yourself about Parkinson's and also learn new ways to care for your loved one.

Find out whether there's a Parkinson's or Parkinson's caregiver support group in your area by checking your local newspaper for community announcements of meetings, or look online for your local Parkinson's chapter, which will be able to tell you about any support groups that may be in your area.

CHAPTER 24
Parkinson's Caregiving: Mid-Stages

The best way out is always through.
~ Robert Frost

Caring for someone with Parkinson's can be both rewarding and challenging. Because Parkinson's progresses at different rates for different people, it's impossible to predict what changes you will face and when you will face them. However, there are things you can do to prepare yourself for the changes that are likely to occur:

Get into a routine

Scheduling is important, especially when it comes to medications and meals. Because some Parkinson's meds must be taken at specific times before and after meals, it's helpful to establish a medication and meal schedule so that it becomes routine.

Plan ahead

As mentioned in chapter 7 on planning, there are several legal documents that you should get drawn up to make sure your loved one gets the kind of care they want in the later stages. These include a HIPAA authorization, a healthcare and financial power of attorney, a living will or advanced care directive, a will, and a trust.

In terms of day-to-day planning, allow extra time for things. For example, when we used to get ready to go shopping with Mom it would take 15 minutes, but as her disease progressed that would sometimes increase to 30 minutes or more.

Speaking of planning ahead, if your loved one is no longer able to drive, you may want to help him or her plan alternative means of transportation. There are several options out there, including public transportation, ride sharing, and community shuttle services.

One thing with respect to planning for mealtimes, especially if your loved one has trouble chewing or swallowing, is that you may want to learn the Heimlich manoeuvre. This is used to dislodge food stuck in the throat if the person is choking, and could be a lifesaver.

Get in tune with medications

As Parkinson's progresses, you will notice inconsistencies in how your loved one reacts to medications. For example, on some days they'll have lots of mobility, and on others not. These "on/off" fluctuations in response to levodopa are common. They may also get more tired than they used to. Because of this, you'll both have to be flexible in your daily planning.

Think about safety concerns

If your loved one's symptoms start to significantly affect their mobility, memory, or thinking skills, you may have to think about whether or not it is safe for them to perform certain daily activities.

For example, driving a car may be dangerous for them, your family, and others on the road. Having to give up driving can be very hard for some people, increasing the burden on the caregiver. You can read more about making decisions about driving in chapter 48.

Don't forget exercise

Exercise, exercise, exercise! You hear all the time – whether you have Parkinson's or not – that regular exercise is important; well, it is. Studies have found that people who begin regular exercise early in the disease experience a slower decline in their quality of life.

Doing 30 minutes of endurance exercise a day maintains muscle control and tone, and also prevents rigidity.

In addition to helping minimize the symptoms of Parkinson's disease, exercise can be emotionally beneficial by helping alleviate depressed or anxious moods.

Just the simple act of getting outside once a day to go for a walk or putter around can loosen up muscles and diminish any depression your loved one might be experiencing.

To help your loved one stay motivated, consider exercising with them. The type of exercise you choose will depend on your loved one's symptoms, fitness level, and overall health. Generally, exercises that stretch the arms and legs through the full range of motion are encouraged.

Some ideas for exercise include walking, swimming, water aerobics (easier on the joints and require less balance), yoga, and tai chi (both of which are relaxing and improve flexibility and balance).

Consider adjusting roles

As Parkinson's progresses, your loved one may no longer be able to take on the same responsibilities or perform the same household tasks they used to. For example, they may have difficulty managing finances, so you may have to take on this role. When it comes to physical tasks like yard work, you may want to consider hiring someone to do that.

Be careful when you go about making these changes, as your loved one may resist or be resentful. Talk things over with them and offer suggestions instead of telling them how things will or will not be.

Get help

As your loved one's Parkinson's progresses, they will have more needs that need to be meet. As a caregiver, you will find that at some point you won't be able meet all these needs. This is where building a caregiver team comes in handy.

The sooner you can start finding outside resources to help you, the better. Look for family or friends who can be your back up in case of an emergency or when you need a break.

Though the people on your caregiving team may play smaller roles for now, having them involved in your loved one's life early on will make it easier for them to fill in for you later when there's a greater need.

Watch for signs of caregiver stress

As Parkinson's progresses and your caregiving role evolves, you may find feelings of regret or resentment creeping in. It's okay to feel this way. Caregiving is a huge job, and especially difficult when you don't see an end in sight.

Throughout your caregiving journey, it's imperative that you care for yourself to make sure that you stay healthy and avoid getting burnt out. You must know and respect your limits. Make it a priority to take regular breaks from caregiving, and when you are with your loved one, look for the things you love about your relationship.

Finally, don't forget that just because your loved one has Parkinson's doesn't mean that they can't take care of you a little. There are many acts of love, including a neck or foot massage, that are pretty easy to deliver through the mid-stages of Parkinson's disease.

CHAPTER 25
Parkinson's Caregiving: Late Stages

Courage isn't having the strength to go on –
it is going on when you don't have strength.
~ Napoleon Bonaparte

QUALITY. This is a word you'll often hear from health care providers as your loved one's Parkinson's advances into the late stages. The reason my mom designated me as POA for her care was because she knew I would do my utmost to make sure she got the best quality of life for as long as she lived. I have taken this role very seriously, and with the help of a "caregiver team," I believe that I've been doing a pretty good job at it.

If you've been caring for a loved one with Parkinson's through to the late stages of the disease, you've probably been serving in your role for a number of years. By now you've also probably experienced how exhausting this job can be, especially when it comes to providing physical care for your loved one.

As Parkinson's progresses into the late stages, you'll find that your loved one's medications become less effective in treating their symptoms. They will need more help with daily activities such as walking, dressing, bathing, and getting in and out of a chair or bed.

In addition to physical challenges, you will notice changes in your loved one's behavior, as well as their thinking and memory.

Even though there are many challenges that accompany advanced Parkinson's, you can still do a lot to make your loved one's life easier, more comfortable, and more enjoyable.

Keep in mind that word – "quality." Focus on making your loved one safe and comfortable. Be patient in this stage and always remember to get help when you need it!

The following chapters in this section will provide the information you need to make things easier for you and your loved one as their Parkinson's progresses.

CHAPTER 26
Home Safety Tips

By changing nothing, nothing changes.
~ Tony Robbins

If you're living in a home with someone with Parkinson's, you'll soon discover that there are various hazards around the house that can make life difficult for them. Fortunately, there are some easy changes you can make to improve their safety.

To begin, start with smaller changes like de-cluttering your home and getting rid of potential obstacles – like scatter rugs and long cords on the floors. Creating a clear path through your home can make mobility so much easier for someone with Parkinson's. The more open spaces you can create between furniture, the better.

The following are some more specific tips to help you make your home safer and "Parkinson's proof":

All rooms

- Add more lights around the house. This can make it easier to navigate at all times of day. Consider touch- or voice-activated lights if these will be easier to turn on and off.

- Create a contrasting pattern on the floor to help your loved one get from A to B more easily. In my mom's case, she had a friend cut out white squares (eight-by-eight inches made of vinyl on one side and sticky material on the other) and tape them to the floor to make a "path" between the kitchen and the bathroom. When Mom needed to get from the kitchen to the bathroom and had trouble walking, she found that looking at the contrasting white squares on the floor helped her brain focus more on getting where she wanted to be. You can also try adding stripes (about a foot apart) to the floor to help with walking.

Bathroom

- Get rid of bath mats that may slip, and add a non-slip mat to the shower or bathtub.
- Install grab bars or safety rails beside or in front of the toilet. You may also want to look into an elevated toilet seat to make standing up easier.
- Install grab bars on the side of the tub to help with getting in and out. Also, install grab bars or portable handles on the shower wall for balance when showering, as well as on the wall beside the toilet.
- If your bathroom has carpet, remove it. Depending on your budget you may also want to consider making it wheelchair accessible (e.g., widening the door, lowering the sink, building a shower that you can roll into with a chair, etc.).

Bedroom

- Put phones or emergency alarm systems in every room.
- Put night-lights in sockets to make it easier to navigate at night.
- Install a pole that stands beside the bed to help your loved one get in and out of it easier. If you can't install a pole because your ceiling is high, you can install a wooden arm or grab bar on the wall. These devices can also help your loved one turn over in bed.
- If the bedroom is currently positioned a long way from the bathroom, you may want to consider moving it closer so as to make getting there that much easier (especially in the middle of the night).

- If it's in your budget, buy a bed with controls for raising and lowering.

Living room

- To avoid slipping and falling, get rid of scatter mats. Also, it is much easier to get around on hardwood or tiled floors than carpet, so you may want to consider replacing your carpets.
- Consider buying adjustable recliners or chairs with straight backs, firm seats, and arm rests. This will make standing easier.
- Install railings along the walls and hallways to help with balance and to prevent falls.
- You may find that having an office chair on wheels in the house is handy as well. If you have hardwood or tiled floors, you can use this as a makeshift wheelchair for someone to push your loved one from A to B.

Outside

- If it's in your budget, consider more significant renovations, such as ramps, stair lifts, and wider doorways.

CHAPTER 27
Helping with Mobility

Start where you are. Use what you have. Do what you can.
~ Arthur Ashe

If you care for someone with Parkinson's, you're most likely already aware of their challenges with mobility. You can help your loved one with this in several ways. The first way is to understand how Parkinson's affects mobility.

When it comes to initiating first steps for walking, a person with Parkinson's may have problems lifting their feet and may have to take a few small and uneasy steps before walking at a steady pace.

In addition, while walking, they may stop swinging their arms. You may also notice them shuffling their feet and walking with their weight on the balls of their feet.

The term "festinant gait" is used to describe when a person starts taking small, short, shuffling steps that become faster and faster. What sometimes happens is that the shuffling becomes so fast that the person falls forward or runs into something.

Sometimes the same happens, only backwards. There was a time when my mom had problems with this. For what seemed like no reason at all, she would start shuffling backwards. We laughed at it so that she would be less anxious, and would say, "Hey, Mom, you need to switch gears, you're in reverse!"

You need to be careful, as the caregiver, if and when you see someone with Parkinson's shuffling because this can lead to falls.

About one-third of people with Parkinson's disease fall relatively frequently and lose their ability to regain their balance when they start to fall, so it is important to stay near them if they're having walking difficulties.

Something called freezing can also happen when a person with Parkinson's is walking. This often happens in doorways, and basically makes it impossible for the person to move. It is like their feet are glued to the ground.

When it comes to increasing mobility with Parkinson's, the first step is to ask your loved one's doctor for an evaluation by a physical therapist. The therapist will draft a detailed evaluation with recommendations for treatment.

Physical therapy can help people who are in various stages of Parkinson's, from the recently diagnosed to those who have had Parkinson's for many years. Though it can't stop the disease, it may help slow the loss of mobility that accompanies Parkinson's.

Physical therapists teach people with Parkinson's disease and their caregivers exercises to increase mobility and describe techniques to deal with specific trouble areas, such as freezing, getting in and out of bed, getting up from a sitting position, etc.

My mom has found physical therapy to be very helpful, and has a physiotherapist visit her once a week. She also tries to get outside every day to go for a walk. This is to help her keep her mobility for as long as possible (remember the statement: "Move it or lose it!").

Sometimes when Mom's mobility isn't great, she pushes her wheelchair to help keep her balance and I (or a friend) walk beside her, there to steady her in case she needs it.

As a caregiver, you will have to pay close attention to what works and what doesn't when it comes to keeping your loved one mobile. Sometimes walking while holding onto you will be better for them than, say, using a walker. One tip to remember is to let them hold onto you more than you hold onto them. This will give your loved one more confidence and allow them to decide when they want to let go.

Something else that Mom has found helpful in terms of increasing her mobility is massage therapy. She loves this and would go all the time if she could afford it!

If your loved one has trouble walking in the house, see if removing all their footwear (including slippery socks) helps. You don't want them wearing shoes that grip the floor and cause them to stumble.

If your loved one has trouble walking through doorways (a common problem for people with Parkinson's disease), suggest that they try walking sideways, a trick that has worked well for Mom.

As mentioned previously, make clear pathways throughout your house to prevent tripping and falling at night. You may also want to install grab bars and railings along the walls, as well as night-lights.

Also mentioned previously was the idea of creating contrasting patterns on the floors. The same principle can be applied outdoors. After we made a stone pathway (made of pre-cut white patio cement that we got at the local hardware store) from the stairs of her house to her garden, Mom was able to "follow the yellow brick road" (or white, in this case) to get to her garden without any problems.

If your loved one is having mobility problems with Parkinson's disease, a contrasting pattern on the floor or ground may be just the thing they need.

CHAPTER 28
Preventing Falls

Act as if what you do makes a difference. It does.
~ William James

Unfortunately, because of the nature of Parkinson's and how it affects balance and stability, people with this disease are prone to falling. Falls become more common as the disease progresses.

In fact, up to two-thirds of people with Parkinson's experience falls each year (compared to a third of the general elderly population).

Falls in Parkinson's occur mostly when turning or changing directions and are often related to a "freezing episode." People with Parkinson's might also experience falls as a result of orthostatic hypotension (postural low blood pressure) and problems with vision.

There is no single solution to preventing falls in Parkinson's disease, and because they become more and more common as people age, the main focus should be on preventing frequent falls and minimizing injury.

As a caregiver, one big thing you can do to help keep your loved one from falling is to make your home safer. Tips on how to do this were mentioned in a previous chapter on home safety for people with Parkinson's.

Here are some more specific tips to help with fall prevention:

- Ensure that your love one takes their medication as prescribed to reduce the severity of motor symptoms.
- Help your loved one stay focused while walking by avoiding distractions. Even talking can contribute to falls, as multitasking may be hard for the Parkinson's brain.

- To increase muscle strength, stability, and balance, have your loved one try an exercise and physical therapy program individually tailored to them.
- Make sure your loved one is wearing appropriate footwear to help them move around more easily and keep them more stable (ladies, put away your heels!). Mom found that walking around barefoot was best for her while in the house.
- Encourage your loved one to always keep one hand free so that they have the other hand to grab onto surrounding objects and/or break the force of a fall if need be.
- Consider withdrawal of psychotropic medications.
- Always seek medical attention, even after a minor fall, to identify the full extent of injuries and have them treated immediately to limit complications.

If your loved one with Parkinson's disease is in a care facility, you may want to consider the following for additional help in preventing falls:

- Use of vitamin D and calcium supplements
- Use of hip protectors

*Note: Studies have shown that there is no evidence to support the effectiveness of interventions to reduce falls among people with cognitive impairments. In addition, using physical or pharmaceutical restraints has not been found to prevent falls. In fact, there is some evidence to support an increased risk of injury from a fall with the use of restraints.

CHAPTER 29
Managing Freezing Episodes

It is not the strength of the body that counts, but the strength of the spirit.
~ J.R.R. Tolkien

One safety challenge many people with Parkinson's, especially those in advanced stages, face is "freezing." Freezing is the temporary, involuntary inability to move. For example, you may find that your loved one's feet seem to stick to the floor, or they may be unable to get up from a chair.

No one knows the exact cause of freezing, but many times this happens when a person is due for their next dose of dopaminergic medications.

Freezing can be dangerous, as it can often lead to falls. As a caregiver, it's very important that you not force someone with Parkinson's disease to walk when they are in this state.

Though you may not always be able to prevent freezing, there are some things you can do to help your loved one through it:

- Encourage your loved one to count their steps as they walk (try marching or "left, right, left, right...").
- One great thing that Mom discovered was music. Try putting on a CD with some fast-paced music to keep them going. Even better, carry an MP3 player (or iPod) with their favorite tunes so they can "plug in" anytime they need a lift.
- Have them rock in place or shift their weight from one foot to another to get moving again.
- Place your foot in front of them, or have them visualize something they need to step over. (You can also use a mobile laser device that creates a line in front of them.)

- Ask them to cover their eyes. This can "trick" their brain and allow them to walk straight ahead with no problems.
- You may choose to simply wait: after all, the freezing will pass.
- If your loved one is in a hurry, they can sink to their knees and crawl, but obviously this is practical only at home.
- Suggest walking very carefully backwards or sideways (this works very well for Mom).

CHAPTER 30
Getting the Most Out of Medications

I'm always trying to find the perfect cocktail of medication and
I think now I've found it.
~ Michael J. Fox

As a caregiver for someone with Parkinson's, you'll soon discover how important medications are in their daily lives. Making sure that they get their medications on time is one of – if not the most – important thing you can do for them throughout their Parkinson's journey. Doing so will give them the best chance of managing their symptoms throughout the day.

Parkinson's medication isn't cheap either, making it very important that your loved one get the most out of each dose.

In addition to getting medications on time, some tips to increase the effectiveness of Parkinson's medications include:

- Take the medication as prescribed by the doctor. Make sure you understand the expected benefit and potential early side effects of a drug before you leave the doctor's office. Remember that he (or she) probably has more clinical experience in treating people with Parkinson's disease than anyone else who is likely to give you advice.
- Do not increase the dosage or suddenly stop the use of any drugs without checking with the doctor.
- Levodopa generally works best on an empty stomach, so aim to take meds around a half hour before meals, or at least an hour after.
- Make sure meds are taken with four to five ounces of water so that the drugs are absorbed into the body more quickly.

- Avoid eating large amounts of protein at any time, as eating too much protein reduces the effectiveness of Parkinson's disease meds.

Though you may not always be able to achieve it, you should aim for as little "off" or "down" time as possible (i.e., time when you are basically staying in one place for a period of time because your medications have worn off).

Some people with Parkinson's find that after they take their meds, there is a period of time before the meds kick in. This is true for my mom. She expects to wait up to 45 minutes (though usually less than this) after she takes her medications for them to start working and for her to have "on" time (or, in her words, for her to "have wheels").

Her way of telling whether or not she is getting the most out of her meds is to see how much time each day she spends in "off" mode. For her, if she has to wait more than an hour for her meds to kick in, or if she spends more than four hours in one day during this down time, she knows that she needs to talk to her doctor about changing the dosage and/or timing of her medications.

One thing that has helped with the effectiveness of her meds is being able to take them on an empty stomach. This wasn't possible for her in the beginning because she got nauseous all the time (a common side effect of the drugs). However, after her body got used to it, she was able to switch the timing of taking her meds.

Mom says that the good thing about having less food in your stomach is that the meds work better. However, sometimes it can seem that they are working too well because you get more of the side effect dyskinesia. You might have to experiment a bit with the timing of meals and meds to find what works best for your loved one.

Another tip Mom has for helping medications work better is to avoid sitting in one place for long lengths of time. If you have to sit anywhere for over an hour at a time, try to get up every hour and do some stretching or moving around to keep your muscles from stiffening up too much. Regardless of when she last took her medications, Mom has found that sitting in one spot for a long time can make it hard to get moving again.

CHAPTER 31
How to Deal with Hallucinations

Fall seven times, stand up eight.
~ Japanese Proverb

Here's something I never knew about Parkinson's when my mom was first diagnosed. People with this disease can experience hallucinations and delusions.

Fortunately, not everyone with Parkinson's experiences these often-frightening symptoms. Those who do are usually older and have had the disease for a long time. Hallucinations and delusions may be caused in part by the disease and in part by the Parkinson's medications.

If you're not sure exactly what a hallucination is, it's when you think that something is there when it isn't. A delusion is when you are convinced that something is true despite clear evidence proving that it is not.

There are different types of hallucinations, including:

- Visual hallucinations (seeing things that aren't there)
- Auditory hallucinations (hearing things that aren't there)
- Tactile hallucinations (sensing things that aren't there)

There are also different types of delusions, including:

- Paranoia (thinking that someone is following you when they aren't)
- Jealousy (thinking that people you love are betraying you)
- Extravagance (believing that you have special powers)

Over the last five years, Mom has had experience with hallucinations, in particular, visual ones. One of the things Mom used to imagine seeing was a big black hole in front of her that she was afraid of falling into. She'd also imagine "a man" (his identity would often change) stealing what she thought were her grandkids.

Through trial and error, we figured out that these hallucinations and delusions were mostly a side effect of a drug (Amantadine) that she takes for her dyskinesia.

At first we tried reassuring her that what she was seeing wasn't real. This helped calm her down initially. However, as the hallucinations got worse and she became more frightened by them, we opted for medication changes.

It is a delicate balance trying to keep her dyskinesia to a minimum while keeping her from having hallucinations. So far, by reducing (not eliminating) the meds she takes for dyskinesia, the hallucinations have stopped.

If your loved one experiences hallucinations or delusions, it's important that you encourage them to talk with you about them. This will help you better support them and understand what they are going through.

If the hallucinations are not frightening and your loved one is aware that they are not real, they may choose to live with this side effect. If, on the other hand, your loved one is frightened, you will want to talk with their doctor to find possible solutions.

The doctor will check for other causes of these symptoms. Things like an imbalance of chemicals in the blood; improper kidney, liver, or lung function; and certain infections can cause these mental disturbances.

Other medications that your loved one may be taking, including over-the-counter medicines, could also be responsible. Make sure that you tell the doctor about all medications, including herbal therapies, that your loved one is taking.

If no other causes for the hallucinations or delusions are found, the doctor may choose to make adjustments to the Parkinson's medications.

Some people may not be able to tolerate changes in their Parkinson's medications without the worsening of their symptoms. In these cases, it may be necessary to treat the mental disturbances with anti-psychotic medicines.

Unfortunately, some of these can worsen Parkinson's disease. There are alternatives, though, and the doctor will be able to help you find them if needed.

CHAPTER 32
How to Handle Weight Loss

Problems are not stop signs, they are guidelines.
~ Robert Schuller

Many people with Parkinson's lose weight after diagnosis. It's a fairly common problem, especially for women. Mom has had issues with this in recent years and it's been a bit of a challenge coming up with the perfect diet to keep her from losing weight.

Researchers aren't entirely sure why this happens. Some think it may be that people with PD eat less due to loss of appetite caused by depression, or loss of sense of smell. Others think it could be all the shaking and dyskinesia associated with the disease or the swallowing problems that cause people with Parkinson's to lose weight.

Whatever the reason behind weight loss in PD, it can have some serious side effects in your loved one, including a weakened immune system, muscle loss, and loss of important nutrients.

If you find your loved one can't stop the weight from coming off, there are several things you can do to can help them.

Consult with their doctor if you think any of the following tips will help:

To help maintain a healthy weight:

- Weigh your loved one once or twice a week, unless your doctor recommends weighing more often. If your loved one is taking diuretics or steroids, you should weigh daily.
- If they have an unexplained weight gain or loss (2 pounds in one day or 5 pounds in one week), talk to your doctor. He or she may want to change food or fluid intake to help manage the condition.

Tips for gaining weight:

- Ask your doctor about nutritional supplements. Sometimes supplements in the form of snacks, drinks (such as Ensure or Boost), or vitamins may be prescribed for consumption between meals to help increase caloric intake and get the right amount of nutrients every day. Mom drinks one Ensure shake a day. Just make sure you look for high-calorie – NOT high-protein – drink supplements. Also, avoid taking medications with these supplements.
- Avoid low-fat or low-calorie products (unless your doctor has recommended otherwise). Use whole milk, whole milk cheese, and yogurt.

*Note: Make sure you check with your doctor before making any dietary changes or before adding supplements to your diet. Some can be harmful or interfere with Parkinson's medications.

To help improve a poor appetite:

- Sometimes poor appetite is due to depression, which can be treated. Talk to your doctor if this applies to your loved one. Their appetite will probably improve after depression is treated.
- Avoid non-nutritious drinks like pop.
- Eat small, frequent meals and snacks.
- Encourage your loved one to walk or get involved in another light activity to stimulate their appetite.

To help eat more at meals:

- Have drinks after a meal instead of before or during a meal to prevent your loved one from feeling full before they start eating.

- Choose foods that are a different color than the plate off which they are eating – people with Parkinson's can develop vision changes, with the amount of contrast sensitivity in the eye making it hard to discern objects that are similar in color. Try using dark-colored dishes when serving light-colored foods and light-colored dishes when serving dark-colored foods.
- Plan meals to include their favorite foods.
- Try eating the high-calorie foods in a meal first.
- Increase the variety of food (use your imagination or a good cookbook).

Tips to help with snacking:

- Choose high-calorie snacks, ideally those with some nutritional value. Examples of these kinds of snacks are: ice cream, cookies, pudding, cheese, granola bars, custard, sandwiches, nachos with cheese, eggs, crackers with peanut butter, bagels with peanut butter or cream cheese, cereal with half and half, fruit or vegetables with dips, yogurt with granola, popcorn with butter and parmesan cheese, and bread sticks with cheese sauce.
- Make food preparation easy. Choose foods that are easy to make and eat.
- Make eating a good experience, not a chore. To liven things up at meal times, try putting on background music and using colorful place settings.
- As much as possible, eat with your loved one so that they aren't eating alone If you're not around for a period of time, encourage them to invite somebody over for dinner or to go out.

CHAPTER 33
Help for Drooling and Dry Mouth

Sometimes singed wings will fly with greater purpose.
~ Tom Althouse

If your loved one has problems with drooling, they may have experienced the embarrassment that it can cause. As their caregiver, you may have felt some of this embarrassment too.

People with Parkinson's appear to have more saliva than people without it because they swallow less often. Drooling is often the result of this excess amount of saliva.

Fortunately, there are some things you can do to prevent drooling. Encourage your loved one to try some of the tips below:

Tips to help drooling:

- Suck on hard candy, lozenges, or gum to control excess saliva (if your loved one is not at risk of choking).
- Use a straw when drinking to strengthen the muscles of the lips, mouth, and throat.
- Try to keep your head up and your posture straight because stooping encourages drooling.
- Swallow first before you talk.
- When you're not eating or talking, keep your mouth closed and your lips tight together (people with PD tend to let their jaws drop open, which encourages drooling).
- Breathe through your nose (this will help keep your mouth closed, which will itself help keep the saliva in your mouth).
- Remind yourself to swallow to help prevent saliva build-up.
- Try rubbing a strong-smelling lip balm over your mouth to remind yourself to swallow.

- Put one or two drops of atropine eye drops (0.5%) under your tongue to reduce the amount of saliva. This works for some people, but you should check with your doctor first.

If nothing else has worked, your loved one may want to consult with their doctor about other alternatives. For example, injections of botulinum toxin (Botox) have been found to help reduce drooling (also called sialorrhea). Doctors inject the Botox into the salivary glands and the effects develop gradually over several days, with the peak reached in about 2 weeks.

The results last about 3 months, so if your loved one chooses this treatment option, they will need to have injections repeated at 3-month intervals to maintain ongoing benefits.

Tips to help dry mouth:

- If not at risk of choking, suck on hard candies or chew gum to help keep your mouth wet/lubricated.
- Try not to eat too many dry foods like peanut butter, crackers, and chips, because they stick to your throat and dry out your mouth.
- Eat sour candy or fruit ice to help increase saliva and moisten your mouth.
- Add sauces (e.g., gravy, broth, sauce, or melted butter) to foods to make them softer and moister.
- Take a drink after each bite of food to moisten your mouth and help you swallow.
- Dunk or moisten bread, toast, cookies, or crackers in milk, tea, or coffee to soften them.
- Breathe through your nose instead of your mouth.
- If your loved one smokes, encourage them to cut down or even quit because this can be a major factor in drying out their mouth and causing gum problems.

- Try taking a cotton swab dipped in olive oil and rubbing it on the inside of your mouth and throat every hour or so.

- Don't use a commercial mouthwash because they often contain alcohol that can dry your mouth; ask your doctor or dentist about alternative mouthwash products.

- Limit caffeine (contained in coffee, tea, cola, and chocolate), as it may make you more thirsty (because caffeine is a diuretic, meaning that it can make you urinate more frequently, resulting in dehydration and increased thirst).

- Consider an artificial saliva product, but ask your doctor about this first.

- Your loved one may need to make changes to their medications.

- Keep hydrated, drinking lots of water (8 glasses a day will help).

*Note: Some people with Parkinson's disease who also have heart problems may need to limit their fluids, so be sure to follow your doctor's guidelines.

CHAPTER 34
Mealtime and Swallowing Tips

Believe you can and you're halfway there.
~ Theodore Roosevelt

Many people with Parkinson's disease have difficulty swallowing because they lose control of their mouth and throat muscles. Because of this, chewing and managing solid foods can be hard.

Problems with swallowing can increase the risk of choking, so it's important as a caregiver that you do as much as you can to learn ways to prevent this.

If your loved one is having trouble swallowing, contact their doctor. He or she can refer you to a speech pathologist who will carefully examine your loved one's swallowing abilities, as well as evaluate and help reduce their risks of choking.

To give you peace of mind, you might want to consider taking a Red Cross course to learn the Heimlich manoeuvre in case of emergency.

Here are some suggestions to make chewing and swallowing easier:

- Sit upright at a 90-degree angle.
- Tilt your head slightly forward.
- Remain sitting or standing for 30 minutes after eating a meal.
- DO NOT give food or medications when lying down.
- Keep distractions to a minimum in the area where you eat.
- Schedule meals during "ON" times – when their medications are working best.
- Stay focused on the tasks of eating and drinking and don't talk with food in your mouth.
- Eat slowly.

- Cut food into small pieces and chew it thoroughly.
- Don't try to eat more than 1/2 teaspoon of your food at a time.
- Swallow two or three times per bite or sip.
- If food or liquid catches in the throat, cough gently or clear your throat, then swallow again before taking a breath. Repeat if necessary.
- Concentrate on swallowing frequently.
- Drink plenty of fluids.
- Periodically suck on popsicles, ice chips, lemon ice, or lemon-flavored water to increase saliva, which will increase how often you swallow.
- Minimize (or eliminate) foods that require chewing, and eat more soft foods.
- Avoid tough, dry, or crumbly textured foods.
- For those who are frequently tired or who feel full quickly, provide small, frequent meals instead of a few big meals.
- Puree foods in a blender.
- If thin liquids cause coughing, thicken them with a liquid thickener (the speech pathologist can recommend one). You can also substitute thin liquids with thicker liquid choices such as nectars for juices and cream soups for plain broths.
- You may want to try a straw to assist in drinking, but use a short one so that they can't take in too much liquid at one time.
- When taking medications, crush the pills and mix them with applesauce. Pudding MAY be okay; however, check the protein content, as it could interfere with the absorption of levodopa.
- ***Note:** Some pills, such as Sinemet CR (controlled release), should not be crushed because this can affect how the medications work. Ask your pharmacist for his/her recommendations on which pills should not be crushed.
- Ask your doctor or pharmacist if your loved one can't swallow medications. Carbidopa-levodopa may also be available as a tablet

that dissolves under the tongue or as a gel that is delivered through a pump to the intestines.

Here are some suggestions to make mealtimes easier:

- Choose a chair that can be pushed all the way under the table so that your loved one can be close to the plate.
- If need be, add pillows to the chair to make it more comfortable.
- There are many adaptive utensils and cups you can buy to help your loved one maintain their independence in eating. These include curved and built-up forks and spoons, rocker knives, plate guards, nosey cups and covered cups. The occupational therapist can help you choose what products would best help your loved one.
- Use an apron or napkin to protect clothes.
- To avoid dehydration, make sure your loved one is getting between 6-8 glasses (48-64 ounces) of liquid per day. To get this daily amount, encourage your loved one to drink a glass of water each time they take their medications. Remember that foods like fruits, vegetables, and ice cream have higher water content, so they can count toward daily fluid intake.

CHAPTER 35
Social Concerns

Being deeply loved by someone gives you strength,
while loving someone deeply gives you courage.
~ Laozi

"My husband had impeccable table manners and even abhorred others that gulped down their food and otherwise expressed poor table etiquette. Now he does things at the table that are downright embarrassing. If I try to correct him, much like a child, he gets offended and angry. But I can't just let him destroy the table and its contents.'
~ Parkinson's Caregiver

Socially speaking, it can be difficult for a person with Parkinson's because others may look at them as though they are, as my mom used to say, some sort of "freak" with all the moving and shaking they do.

In reality, most people probably don't look at people with Parkinson's as freaks, but it's easy to feel that way when you have the disease.

As the disease progresses, it can sometimes be hard to be in public. For instance, when my mom would experience a sudden shutdown of her body, she would often have trouble walking through doorways. This would then attract attention from others, and was emotionally disturbing for her.

Also, it can sometimes be hard for a person with PD to eat out because they can have trouble holding onto cutlery. Several times, my mom would get embarrassed and upset because she couldn't stop dropping things at the dinner table. Even amongst friends, she often found eating very emotionally difficult.

Finally, Parkinson's can be hard on your social life, especially if you have a partner with PD who can no longer do the things (like going out dancing) you used to do. Finding new activities that you both can do together is the key here. Remember not to let Parkinson's get between the two of you!

With all this said, as a caregiver of someone with Parkinson's, it's important that you understand how they feel, and do your best to support and reassure them.

When you're in public, try to ignore any unwanted attention your loved one may be receiving. This may be hard for both of you at first, but over time you will develop ways to deal with different social situations.

Sometimes when Mom and I were out shopping, I would tell the salesperson about Mom having Parkinson's. Every time I did, we received nothing but help and empathy. You may or may not choose to do this, but I have found most people are afraid of what they don't know, so helping them understand a bit about Parkinson's helps.

--- ~ ---
PART 6
ESPECIALLY FOR SPOUSES
--- ~ ---

CHAPTER 36
Special Needs of Spousal Caregivers

Will you still need me, will you still feed me, when I'm sixty-four.
~ The Beatles, *"When I'm 64"*

"In sickness and in health…" As a spousal caregiver, this vow may mean a lot more than you ever thought it would. If so, you may feel better knowing that there are millions of others out there just like you. According to the National Family Caregivers Association, over half of all caregivers in America are caring for a spouse.

Caring for a spouse with Parkinson's can be emotionally draining and stressful. It can be hard shifting from spouse to caregiver and you may not know how to deal with the challenges that come with the new role.

You may also have to deal with feelings of loneliness in your relationship, of isolation from friends, and resentment or anger toward your spouse. If your loved one has dementia in addition to Parkinson's, you may also have to deal with a sense of loss.

With all this on your plate, it's imperative that you make sure your needs are being met. In fact, caring for yourself can be one of the most important things you to do help your loved one. It can help you maintain your marriage while you shift into the caregiver role, and also help prevent stress and burnout, which will enable you to provide better care.

Failing to take care of your needs can lead to a decline in your own health and even increase your risk of death. Studies have found that spousal caregivers have a significantly higher risk (over 60 percent) of dying than do their non-caregiving peers if they experience ongoing mental and emotional strain.

There are many ways to take care of yourself, and we will discuss these in more detail throughout the rest of the book. Two key things to remember are to allow others to help you (caregiving is not a solo job) and to take regular breaks.

CHAPTER 37
What to Do When Your Life Becomes All About Parkinson's

To thine own self be true.
~ William Shakespeare, *Hamlet*

"My husband has had Parkinson's disease for 11 years. He is 58 years old and getting into advanced stages now. All our life is Parkinson's. About how he doesn't sleep and his foot cramps. All his medicine he has to take. That's most our conversations and it's getting very depressing for me. I have tried to tell him to talk about something different and now I have given up on this matter. It wears me down. Please help!" ~ Parkinson's Caregiver

Unfortunately, the previous sentiments expressed by a Parkinson's caregiver are quite common. If you've been caring for your loved one for some time, Parkinson's can end up consuming your life. This is especially common among spousal caregivers, as they spend most, if not all, of their time with their loved one.

If you've found yourself in a situation in which Parkinson's is taking over, there are steps you can take to regain balance in your life:

Know yourself

Caregiving is something you *do* – it is not meant to define who you *are*. Though caregiver may be one of your roles, it's important to realize and remind yourself that you have other roles as well. In my case, I am also a wife, a daughter, a sister, an aunt, a friend, a swimmer, and a writer, among other things.

If you dig deeper you'll find I'm sensitive and empathetic to those in need (in particular the elderly), and I tend to wear my heart on my sleeve. I'm also analytical, super competitive, and very passionate about a lot of things.

Take some time to think about who you are and the roles you play in your life. Knowing yourself will enable you to figure out what your limits are, as well as decide what you feel comfortable with and how much you are willing to give in your caregiving role.

Set boundaries

As a spouse caring for someone with Parkinson's, there may be assumptions that you do everything. Friends, family, even doctors and nurses may say, "Don't worry, the wife/husband will do it." Sometimes people assume that because you're the spouse, you should be prepared and willing to do everything that needs to be done.

It's okay to express that you're completely overwhelmed in your caregiving role. We all have limits, and as a spousal caregiver, you don't – and shouldn't – have to do it all.

Setting boundaries with which you are comfortable is an important step in ensuring that you are able to be the best caregiver you can be. Talk to your spouse about how you're feeling, and in a loving and caring way discuss what you are and aren't willing and able to do.

Set goals

It's easy to put your life on hold while you're immersed in a caregiving role. The problem is that you probably won't know how long your life will be on hold. In the meantime, you could lose out on many opportunities.

Having goals can help make life more exciting and give you something to strive for. To help you achieve your goals, make sure you are consistently working on them. Even if it's for only 15 minutes a day, you'll find that your goals gain momentum if you stick with them consistently over time.

Reconnect with your spouse

It's easy for a marriage to get lost in Parkinson's. To reconnect in your marriage, allow yourself to just *be* with your partner instead of focusing on what needs to be done all the time.

If you find this hard to do, consider giving up caregiving tasks that may be more demanding or that cause stress in your relationship. Hiring someone to come in to take the load off you can enable you to focus on spending more quality time with your spouse.

CHAPTER 38
When Parkinson's is
Keeping You Up All Night

A good laugh and a long sleep are the best cures in the doctor's book.
~ Irish Proverb

Parkinson's disease creates many challenges with respect to getting a good night's sleep. In fact, it has been estimated that almost 90 percent of those with PD experience sleep difficulties of some kind.

If you're caring for a spouse with Parkinson's, their sleep problems will most likely affect the quality of your sleep as well.

These sleep problems can include insomnia, disrupted sleep, hallucinations, nightmares, vivid dreaming, sleepwalking, sleep talking, sleep apnea (when breathing stops for a few seconds), excessive daytime sleepiness (EDS), nocturia (waking up with the urge to urinate), and restless leg syndrome (RLS).

There are many possible reasons for sleep problems in people with PD. One of the more common ones is medication. People with Parkinson's often have problems falling or staying asleep when PD meds (e.g., Levodopa or other Dopamine agonists) start to wear off before the next dose is due. This causes symptoms such as tremor, rigidity, pain, and turning over in bed.

The anti-Parkinson's medications Amantadine and Selegiline can also make it hard for people to fall or stay asleep, due to their stimulant effect. My mom has had this problem. With advanced Parkinson's she can sometimes experience excessive dyskinesia, for which she takes Amantadine to control. Though the Amantadine does work to calm her body down, it unfortunately also tends to keep her awake, sometimes for the entire night.

Anxiety, depression, and other psychological problems (including dementia) are also causes of insomnia and sleep disturbances.

Other medications can be responsible for sleep disruptions. Diuretics (tablets to promote urine production and flow) can be at fault because if you don't take them early enough, you may have to get up a lot during the night to go to the bathroom.

The drug ephedrine (a stimulant used to treat postural hypotension) can also disrupt sleep, so be aware of this. Don't forget that over-the-counter pills like decongestants or antihistamines may cause sleep problems as well.

Many people forget that food is often at fault. Stay away from stimulants, especially caffeine. Caffeine is found in such things as tea and chocolate, as well as coffee. Alcohol may initially make you tired but can ultimately be a stimulant, causing you to wake up early in the morning.

As a spouse, you can help your partner by learning more about their individual problems with sleep and consulting with their doctor to find ways to improve their quality and quantity of sleep.

Here are some tips that may help your spouse have more comfortable, restful sleep:

For problems moving or turning in bed:

- Try side rails, a trapeze, ropes, or a handle to grip.
- Use satin sheets and pajamas – NOT flannel ones, as they make rolling and moving in bed difficult (Mom says satin sheets are the best!).
- Change to a firmer, lower mattress. DON'T use waterbeds or soft mattresses, as they may make moving in bed much harder.
- Ask a physical therapist, as they may be able to help with bed mobility. Occupational therapists may recommend other techniques.

For foot and leg sensitivity in bed:

- Adapt the bed with a bed hoop, blanket cradle, electric blanket, or light down comforter in order to keep the bedcovers off feet and legs.

For restless legs, painful cramping, or abnormal movements:

- Talk to their doctor because he or she might change the times or dosages of your spouse's medications, or order other medications for pain, spasm, cramps, or anxiety.
- Try some relaxation techniques or slow, relaxing stretching exercises.
- Walk around to help relieve restless leg syndrome (RLS).

For frequent urination at night:

- Talk to their doctor or urologist to correct medical problems such as prostate problems, urinary retention, or infections.
- Put a urinal or commode near the bedside.

For reducing the risks of falling at night:

- Make your home safer by getting rid of scatter rugs and putting in a nightlight.
- Suggest that your spouse use a walker at night if they are able to do so.
- Tell your spouse not to get up too quickly or they might become dizzy from changing position too quickly.
- Make sure the bed is low enough so that your spouse can get their feet on the floor easily (removing bed casters can help with this).
- DON'T use high mattresses that require the assistance of a step stool or platform to get onto.

For shortness of breath, heartburn, or trouble getting out of bed:

- Raise the head of the bed with blocks or extra pillows.
- Discuss shortness of breath and heartburn with their doctor.
- Use hand rails or a bed pole for leverage to make getting in and out of bed easier.

Another tip you may want to consider is sleeping in side-by-side twin beds, or even in separate rooms, to ensure better rest for both of you. If you decide to sleep in separate rooms, your loved one could use a call button, alert system, or monitor to let you know if they need help.

CHAPTER 39
How Can I Regain Respect for My Spouse With PD?

I don't want someone who sees the good about me.
I want someone who sees the bad and still loves me.
~ Unknown

"How can I get the respect back that I had for my husband before he became ill with Parkinson's? With his constant dribbling and incontinence issues I do struggle even though I know that it is not his fault. Luckily I am able to still leave him on his own some times during the day to regain my sanity but as soon as I return, the feeling returns. I hate myself for feeling this way."
~ Parkinson's Caregiver

When your role of wife or husband has shifted to caregiver, there are many challenges you will face, including some that may be difficult for you to admit. Losing respect for the person you married is one challenge that can arise, especially in the later stages of the disease.

If you're struggling with this, don't beat yourself up about it. Recognizing when your feelings toward your spouse have changed can spur you on to take steps toward regaining respect for them.

Though it may not always be easy, there are some things you can do to let your spouse know you still respect them:

- Know it's not their fault. Remember that it is Parkinson's – NOT them – that is making your spouse act or feel a certain way.
- Find something you respect about your spouse. Even if it is something as small as your spouse smelling nice, let them know you respect that about them and affirm them in those areas.
- Show them love and affection. Remember that your spouse is not Parkinson's. Though they may have symptoms that neither of

you enjoy, they are still the person you married and need you to be close to them when they are suffering.

- Know and accept your spouse's limitations. Living with Parkinson's can be frustrating and depressing at times. Don't make things worse by unintentionally setting up your spouse for failure by expecting them to do things they can't do.

- Educate yourself about Parkinson's. Parkinson's affects every aspect of life, so the more you know, the more supportive and compassionate you can be toward your spouse.

- Avoid dwelling on what could have been. Nothing in life is for certain, so accept your situation and make the best of it. Look for and talk about the things for which you are thankful. Find things you can both look forward to and set reachable goals together.

- Communicate openly. Encourage your spouse to talk about his or her feelings. What does your spouse need more or less of? Let them know what your needs are as well.

- Avoid scolding and criticizing your spouse. Good things never come from doing either of these.

- Don't patronize or talk down to them. This sometimes happens when a loved one develops dementia and starts behaving like someone much younger than they are. Resist doing this; instead, be kind and reassuring.

- Respect your spouse's privacy, and be sensitive if they need help with personal activities like washing or going to the toilet.

- Take a break together. Find a mutual interest outside of Parkinson's, something you can both enjoy, and do it! It could be something as simple as going for a walk, reading together, or watching a funny movie at home. Having a life together outside of Parkinson's will make your marriage both stronger and happier.

- Know that it's okay to get emotional. It's not easy to live with and care for a spouse with Parkinson's and it may cost you a lot of emotional energy. Give yourself permission to feel the things you are feeling as you face caregiving challenges. Find a friend or professional to whom you can talk when you're feeling overwhelmed, frustrated, angry, or sad. This will help you stay emotionally healthy and in the best shape to support your spouse.

CHAPTER 40
Parkinson's and Your Sex Life

We waste time looking for the perfect lover,
instead of creating the perfect love.
~ Tom Robbins

Many spouses caring for someone with Parkinson's have difficulties talking about the topic of sex, and for good reason – it's a sensitive and sometimes uncomfortable and embarrassing subject.

As you've been caring for your loved one with PD, you may or may not have encountered problems that the disease can cause with respect to your sex life. Some sexual problems your spouse may experience include a decreased sex drive, an increased or "hyper" sexuality, or difficulties with arousal.

Having a lower sex drive may be caused by the decreased dopamine in Parkinson's brains, but it more likely has to do with factors like the stress, anxiety, and depression that can result after diagnosis rather than it being a direct result of Parkinson's.

Though it may be less romantic, you may need to do a little planning before being intimate, or possibly look at different ways of doing so.

On the opposite end of the spectrum are those with PD who experience hyper sexuality. This is a type of impulsive and compulsive behavior in which people find themselves preoccupied with sexual feelings and thoughts.

Hyper sexuality can be a side effect of dopamine agonists (and sometimes levodopa), so if it becomes an issue, a change of meds may be needed. Ask your spouse's doctor to see what may be best for your situation.

Another sexual problem people with PD often have is with arousal. For men, erectile dysfunction is a common problem. Of course, erection problems are common in men as they age, but men with Parkinson's can have even more trouble with this, as the disease negatively impacts the central nervous system, circulation, and muscle function. Again, consulting with the doctor can help you both address this.

--- ~ ---
PART 7
GETTING HELP
--- ~ ---

CHAPTER 41
Respite Care

In the midst of movement and chaos, keep stillness inside you.
~ Deepak Chopra

Respite. If you plan on being a caregiver for any length of time, get used to this word. Respite is defined as "a short period of rest or relief from something difficult or unpleasant."

Respite care means taking a break from caregiving, usually because someone else is taking care of your loved one for a few hours, days, or weeks.

You may hear some people saying that you're "running away," but you're not. You're just stepping off the playing field for a little bit and giving yourself a break. This can also be a good break for your loved one with PD.

As the needs of the care receiver will vary, so will the amount of time off a caregiver will need. Depending on how much care your loved one needs on a daily basis, you may find that taking a few 15-20 minute breaks throughout the day is enough. Some caregivers need more than this, however, and choose to take one or multiple days off a week in order to avoid burnout.

Remember, as a caregiver it's important that you not feel guilty about wanting to have time off and have a respite worker come in. It's not selfish for you to want this time off. Rather, it is absolutely necessary that you take it, for both your sake and the sake of the person for whom you are caring.

Help can come from many people, including friends, family, neighbors, or respite workers from local organizations. A respite worker is someone who comes into your home and helps a person with PD with the activities of daily living, cooking, house cleaning, etc.

When you're looking for formal respite care in your community, you should find several types available. These include companions, homemakers, home health aides, adult day care, and overnight care for a few days or longer in a facility such as a nursing home.

Two types of formal respite care that have proven themselves valuable to caregivers are described below:

Adult Day Care

Many people think that adult day care is just a nicer way of describing what is essentially a nursing home. This is not true. Adult day care programs work to help people keep their independence longer by offering activities and services geared toward their needs, knowledge, abilities, and level of participation.

Some activities offered at adult day care centers may include:

Arts and crafts
Exercise classes
Musical entertainment and sing-a-longs
Mental stimulation games such as bingo and board games
Discussion groups (books, films, current events)
Holiday and birthday celebrations
Local outings
Occupational therapy
Massage therapy

Adult day care programs are offered in a safe and secure environment, and most provide a light breakfast, lunch, and snacks. Some even have support and counseling services for caregivers, and provide transportation to and from your home.

If your loved one needs extra care, supervision, or companionship during the day, or if you're in need of respite during daytime hours, adult day care centers may be the solution for you.

The costs for these programs vary depending on where you live and what services they provide (e.g., meals, transportation, nursing supervision), but in the U.S. they average about $64 a day.

Where there are professional health services, higher fees will apply. Some facilities offer their services on a sliding scale, meaning that what you pay is based on your income and ability to pay. In addition, if you have a very low income, Medicaid may pay for most if not all of the costs.

You can find adult day care programs through your doctor or local aging society or by searching online for Adult Day Care, Aging Services, or Senior Citizen's Services.

Home Health Care

Another popular formal respite choice is home health care. Home health care provides a wide range of health care services in your home. This type of service is usually less expensive, more convenient, and just as effective as the care you would get in a skilled nursing facility.

There are many reasons you may want to use home health care services as part of respite. One reason is for you to get relief from the more physically and emotionally draining caregiving tasks, such as bathing, toileting, and dressing. This will help prevent burnout.

Another reason is having the convenience of being able to leave your home while the health care worker is there with your loved one, and having the choice to pay for only the hours or services you need (anywhere from a couple of hours to a whole day).

Your loved one may also appreciate home care if they have lost their ability to drive. A home care worker can provide transportation and accompany your loved to run errands or go to social events.

Finally, hiring a home care worker can give you peace of mind. Knowing that your loved one is getting the care they need when you're not around can really ease your worries. This type of care comes in really handy if you live apart from your loved one and are caregiving from a distance.

Rates for home health care vary depending on where you live and the amount of care you will need. In the U.S., the average cost of home care per hour ranges between $10 and $36.

If you live in the U.S., one good online resource for finding home care is Senior Helpers. They have recently partnered with the Michael J. Fox Foundation to create home health care services specifically for people with Parkinson's. They also provide in-home services for those with Alzheimer's and dementia.

You can learn more about them by visiting their website: www.seniorhelpers.com.

You can also find resources online by doing a search for Home Health Care in your state/province.

If you're unsure about whether or not this type of care is for you and your loved one, the following questions may help you decide if Home Care is an option:

1. Can your loved one's basic needs be met in the available space? The house may need to accommodate large assistive devices such as a lift-chair, walker, wheelchair, bedside toilet, etc.

2. If you are the primary caregiver, do you work at home or need to be away from the home many hours during the day? If so, hiring outside help may be advisable. Someone must be available and willing to give medications at the scheduled times, prepare meals, assist with personal care, and provide transportation and companionship.

3. Do you have the physical and emotional strength to manage the care needs of your loved one? If not, hiring outside help may be the best option for you.

4. Is the physical layout of the home user-friendly for your loved one? Small doorways, stairs, and bathrooms are just three areas

you will have to look at in your home to decide whether or not Home Care would be an option. There are modifications that should be made in advance to ensure the space is safe and comfortable (ramps at entryways, handrails, bathroom modifications, etc.).

5. Are there limitations such as young children in the home or lack of financial resources that need to be considered? These could both contribute to a less-than-happy living environment.

6. Does your loved one want to live with family members or would they prefer a formal care facility? Make sure you take into consideration your loved one's wishes.

If and when you decide to look for extra care inside your home there are several potential options, depending on how much care you want (visiting or live-in) and what kind of budget you have.

Whatever type of caregiver you choose, you'll want to make sure you screen them by hiring a company to do a background check and to check their credentials.

CHAPTER 42
Housing Options

I find the great thing in this world is, not so much where we stand,
as in what direction we are moving.
~ Goethe

If you're new to the Parkinson's caregiving journey, thinking of where your loved one will live as their disease progresses may not be remotely on your mind. Even if you have thought about it, there's been no question – they'll live with you at home!

Of course, you may decide that your loved one will live with you for the duration of their disease, but for some who find the caregiving load in the later stages of Parkinson's to be too heavy, there are several alternatives to consider.

Before looking at the different types of senior housing available, it's a good idea to take stock of your loved one's care needs. Determining what daily activities they need help with will help you discern the type of housing that will best suit them.

There are two main categories of daily activities that aging adults (and, likewise, people with Parkinson's) typically need assistance with:

1. Instrumental Activities of Daily Living (IADLs)

These activities deal with the day-to-day maintenance of a person's environment:

Cooking
Doing laundry
Housekeeping
Driving
Financial management
Medication management

Using the telephone

2. Basic Activities of Daily Living (BADLs)

These activities involve attending to a person's hygiene, mobility, and bodily care needs:

Bathing

Dressing

Toileting

Eating

Walking/getting up

Once you've discerned what activities your loved one needs help with, the next step is to learn about the various housing choices available.

Many people get overwhelmed at this point, as there are many options. To make things easier, we've described these choices and listed the pros and cons of each:

Living at Home/"Aging in Place"

This is self-explanatory; your loved one lives at home or with a close relative while their disease progresses.

As mentioned in the previous chapter, Adult Day Care centers can be a great option if your loved one is living at home, offering many activities for them while creating a caregiving break for you. Also, home care agencies can make things a lot more convenient for you by coming to your home and providing needed care for your loved one.

PROS:

- Many aging adults feel best about living at home.
- Family members feel good about not putting their loved one in a nursing home.
- Care can be provided by either family members or home care professionals.

CONS:

- Being the primary caregiver can be very emotionally, physically, and financially demanding.
- Caring for a loved one with Parkinson's can be a long journey, requiring you to give many years of your life.
- Relationships with your loved one may become strained.

Independent Living/ Retirement Communities

Independent Living communities offer various types of accommodations, from apartment-style living to freestanding homes.

Other names for Independent Living:
55+ Communities
Active Adult Communities
Adult Lifestyle Communities
Life-Lease Communities
Retirement Homes
Senior Apartments
Seniors Housing

PROS:

- If your loved one is ready to move into a senior living community and is still able to care for themselves, Independent Living communities may provide the freedom and socialization they need.

CONS:

- Some communities provide assistance with certain BADLs (transportation, light housekeeping), but most aren't equipped to care for someone who needs extra help with bathing, dressing, etc.

Assisted Living

Assisted living is good for those aging adults who want to keep their independence but who need help with some of their daily activities, such as meal preparation and/or bathing.

Assisted living areas include one-bedroom apartments, studios with or without kitchenettes, and single or shared rooms.

Other names for Assisted Living:
Congregate Care
Independent Supportive Living
Retirement Care
Supportive Housing

PROS:
- If your loved one isn't safe living alone and needs only minimal assistance, assisted living may be a good option for them.
- Staff is available to help with Instrumental Activities of Daily Living (IADLs), and medical professionals are there 24/7 in case your loved one's needs increase.

CONS:
- As staff will be supervising your loved one when you're not there, the tradeoff is that your loved one will likely lose some of their overall sense of independence.
- The cost of assisted living does not normally include assistance with IADLs or BADLs. These services are available, but they will add to the price, so make sure you ask upfront what's included and what's not.

Skilled Nursing Facility (SNF)/Nursing Home

A skilled nursing facility/nursing home normally offers the highest level of care for aging adults outside of a hospital. They are designed for those who need round-the-clock, 24-hour care.

PROS:
- Skilled nursing facilities/nursing homes have come a long way in recent years, and many are working hard to lose their negative image and to help elders live with dignity.
- The services of nurses, doctors, and physical, occupational, and speech therapists are all offered in SNF/nursing homes.

CONS:
- Your loved one may lose a lot of their freedom and independence.
- As a family member or caregiver, you may feel guilty for putting your loved one in a home.

Continuing Care Retirement Community (CCRC)

The CCRC is a fairly new type of senior housing. It is designed to allow your loved one to remain within the same community, but move into higher levels of care as their needs change.

PROS:
- CCRC's may be a good option for your loved one if they want stability and security, as CCRC's take a lot of the unknowns out of the future.
- Your loved one can more easily transition from one care level to the next without the stress or hassle of moving to a completely new environment.

- There are a wide range of healthcare services provided, which may include nursing, doctor's care, social work, physical therapy, speech therapy, occupational therapy, a pharmacy, dietary assistance, and more.
- CCRC's offer many organized social and physical activities tailored to seniors' tastes. They are also most often situated in peaceful surroundings.

CONS:

- CCRC's aren't cheap. Depending on where you live, this type of housing can be the most expensive long-term care option for your loved one. In most cases, residents are required to pay a large entrance fee, then a monthly fee after that. In some cases, residents buy the unit but still pay a monthly fee for services.
- It can be confusing to navigate the various types of complex contracts. It will be important to have an elder law attorney look over your contract to make sure you know what your loved one is signing up for.
- Administrators have the last word when it comes to when your loved one will move from one level of care to the next.

CHAPTER 43
When is it Time to Apply for Disability?

Tisn't life that matters! It's the courage you bring to it.
~ Hugh Walpole

If your spouse or parent has Parkinson's and they are employed, how long they are able to work will most likely affect you as well. Because of this, the decision of if and when to apply for disability is something you may want to discuss together so that you can be sure to make the right choice.

Because every case of Parkinson's is different, the decision won't be the same for everyone. Generally speaking, if you live in the U.S., your loved one with PD will be eligible to file for a disability application the day after they stop working or the day after their earnings drop below $1,130 per month (the SGA level as of 2016).

If you believe your loved one is disabled and unable to work, and also believe that you may qualify for disability benefits, you should probably minimize the waiting time by filing a Social Security disability or SSI application as soon as you are eligible. It is not uncommon for an application to take 6-8 months to complete despite the "estimated" 90-120 days that the Social Security Administration says it will take.

However, if your loved one's Parkinson's disability isn't obvious or doesn't show clear-cut long-term impairment, some disability attorneys suggest that they wait until they haven't worked for six months before they apply for benefits.

Then, if your initial claim is denied, you have to go through the appeal process, which adds even more time to the whole equation.

Given these conditions, claimants for Social Security disability or SSI benefits often find themselves in great financial distress prior to a disability hearing.

The following links can give you more detailed information on applying for disability:

If you live in the U.S.:

www.ssa.gov/disability/

www.disability.gov/what-is-the-difference-between-social-security-disability-insurance-and-supplemental-security-income/

If you live in Canada:

www.canada.ca/en/services/benefits/disability.html

If you live in Australia:

www.australia.gov.au/information-and-services/benefits-and-payments/people-with-disability

If you live in the U.K.:

www.gov.uk/financial-help-disabled/overview

CHAPTER 44
How Can We Pay for Caregiving Costs?

Perseverance is not a long race; it is many short races one after the other.
~ Walter Elliot

We had to sell our family cottage on Canning Lake to pay for Mom's nursing home costs. My grandpa built the cottage, and all of us – Mom, her four kids, her grandkids, our cousins, even our second cousins – grew up having the most magical, never-ending summers there.

It was such a special place, our family vowed to keep it in the family forever and never sell it…until we had to.

Losing the cottage was one of the biggest losses I've experienced in my life.

At first I was angry at Parkinson's for taking my mom from us, and then for taking our beloved cottage. Then I got angry at "the system" for requiring us to pay so much money for Mom to be taken care of.

If you've been on a Parkinson's journey with a loved one for any length of time, you may be able to relate to our story. At the minimum, you've probably had to take a look at your finances and financial future.

For the record, I want to say that although I was very sad about losing the cottage, in the end I have been very thankful that we had an asset we could liquidate so as to pay for Mom's care. The money we made off the sale of that cottage will cover about 8 years of nursing home costs.

Another reason I'm thankful is that Mom lives in Canada, where nursing home costs are considerably more affordable than they are in the U.S. Wherever you live, it's a good idea to have a long-term plan to pay for care costs.

As you begin to plan for paying for care costs, there are several avenues you can go down. To start, it is possible that your loved one may qualify for financial help from your government. It is very important that you investigate this to see if you qualify because there are many ways in which the government might be able to help you and your loved one.

Depending on what country you live in, you may receive more or fewer benefits.

Some governments provide help to buy things like wheelchair ramps, or help in providing funding to renovate your house to make things easier for you. In most cases, you pay part of the amount, and the government pays the other.

Some governments (e.g., the U.S.) have established or authorized some type of program to provide pharmaceutical (as in prescribed medication) coverage for low-income seniors or people with disabilities who do not qualify for Medicaid, or their federal health benefits program.

Many governments will offer income tax relief to people with Parkinson's. You will need to fill out forms to apply for this, but it's definitely worth checking into to see if your loved one qualifies.

Sometimes, applying for benefits can be complicated, time-consuming, and frustrating. Two things you need to remember when going through this process are: 1) do not throw away any potentially relevant paperwork you receive from an employer, an insurer, a government agency, or an advocate on your behalf, and 2) keep copies of everything you submit.

Outside of government funding, there aren't many organizations that give straight cash. Well, not that we could find, anyway. (If you know of some, let us know!)

One non-government organization we found that does help is called The Melvin Weinstein Parkinson's Foundation. This a non-profit organization dedicated to purchasing the equipment and health supplies necessary to maintain a safe and healthy environment for Parkinson's patients. With the aid of support groups, they locate Parkinson's patients who have financial and medical needs, and find a way to help them. To find out more, check out their website: www.mwpf.org.

The best way to receive monetary support is through employment disability benefits (see the previous chapter for information about that), or various federal health and/or disability support plans.

If you have a low income and few assets other than your home, you may be eligible for Medicaid health care coverage. This includes in-home care and personal care, such as help with bathing, dressing, cooking, cleaning, eating, moving around, and similar activities of daily living.

But before you do this, remember that there are planning options that you can use to make the most of your assets. For help, you should consult a knowledgeable elder law attorney in your state. You can find one through the National Academy of Elder Law Attorneys.

If possible, work with someone who is a certified elder law attorney (CELA). Remember, it is important to get a referral to make sure you find an attorney with whom you are comfortable.

As was said before, you will need to do some research to find out whether or not you qualify for government assistance. You might start with your local chapter for Parkinson's (you can find them online), and they can tell you where you need to go.

Here are a few other online financial resources you may find helpful:

If you live in the U.S.:

www.payingforseniorcare.com

If you live in Canada:

www.aplaceformom.com/canada/how-to-pay-for-senior-housing

If you live in Australia:

www.humanservices.gov.au/customer/subjects/payments-older-australians

If you live in the U.K.:

www.carehome.co.uk/
www.housingcare.org/elderly-uk-nursing-homes.aspx

www.careuk.com/care-homes/

Medicaid (U.S.)

www.healthcare.gov

www.healthcare.gov/do-i-qualify-for-medicaid

Benefits Checkup (U.S.)

www.benefitscheckup.org

Benefits Checkup is the nation's most comprehensive Web-based service to screen for benefits programs for seniors with limited income and resources.

Government Benefits

GovBenefits.gov is the official benefits website of the U.S. government, with information on more than 1,000 benefit and assistance programs.

National Academy of Elder Law Attorneys:

www.naela.org

--- ~ ---

PART 8
CARING FOR *YOU*

--- ~ ---

CHAPTER 45
Putting On the Oxygen Mask

Out of clutter, find simplicity. From discord, find harmony.
In the middle of difficulty lies opportunity.
~ Albert Einstein

If you've been a caregiver for any length of time, you've probably read or heard about the "oxygen mask thing." If you haven't heard this analogy before, let me quickly explain.

When you fly on a plane there's a mandatory safety briefing you receive from the flight attendants prior to takeoff. The speech isn't that exciting, but it contains a very important recommendation: "In the event of a change in air pressure, please put on your own oxygen mask before assisting the person next to you."

When you hear this for the first time, your immediate response is, "No way, I need to take care of my kids (husband, mother, best friend, etc.) first!" The idea opposes your instincts.

The problem with this thinking is that if you don't put on your mask first, you won't be there for those who need you – you'll be unconscious.

The same applies to caregivers. Because we love and care so much, we often focus all our attention on our loved one and neglect to take care of ourselves. However, just like the oxygen mask, we need to take care of ourselves so that we can effectively take care of our loved ones.

Here are some tips to help you take better care of yourself:

Decide that your life matters

It's easy to get consumed with caring for your loved one, even to the point of feeling like you have to be "on call" all the time. Though it may be hard to do, you must realize that you deserve time to yourself to regain peace and calm in your life.

Deciding that your life matters just as much as your loved one's life does is the first step toward taking better care of yourself and making the most of your time away from them.

Take responsibility for your own care

You can't control Parkinson's and how it will affect your loved one. You can, however, take control of your own care.

Contrary to what you might think, focusing on your needs while being a caregiver is not selfish – it's actually an important part of the job. Don't forget – YOU are responsible for taking care of yourself.

There are many things you can do to take control of your own care:

- Make sure you're getting enough rest.
- Pay attention to your nutrition.
- Exercise regularly (even if it's for only 15 minutes at a time).
- Learn to look for and accept other people's help and support.
- Learn and use stress-reduction techniques (e.g., meditation, prayer, yoga, or Tai Chi).
- Take time off (without feeling guilty).
- Find ways to nurture your body and soul (e.g., taking a hot bath or reading a good book).
- Talk to a friend, counselor, or pastor about your feelings when you need to.
- Reduce negativity in your life.

Reduce your stress levels

There are several factors that influence stress levels in any caregiving situation. Stress is not just influenced by the situation itself, but also be how you perceive it.

For example, some naturally see the glass as half full while others see it as half empty. Remembering that you're not the only one going through your experiences may help you see and cope with things differently.

Other factors may influence your stress levels; one of these factors is whether or not your caregiving job was voluntary. If you feel that you had no choice in taking on the responsibility, it's more likely that you'll feel resentful toward your loved one and experience tension in your relationship.

Another factor that can influence your stress levels is the amount of care your loved one needs. For instance, caring for someone with dementia is often more stressful than for someone who has only physical limitations. Your stress levels can be exacerbated if you have little to no support.

Reducing your stress levels is possible by learning some techniques (described in detail in Chapter 11). As you're doing this, think about whether or not you were able to cope with stress in the past, and how you did it.

Set goals

As mentioned earlier in this book, setting goals is a key part of taking care of yourself. If you've never set goals before, think of it as writing a list of things you need to get done.

Start with a list of things you would like to accomplish in the next month, then 3 months, then 6 months. Set small and big goals. Break the big goals down into smaller action steps. This will increase your likelihood of accomplishing them. Also, the more specific you can be with your goals, the better.

Some examples of goals you might set are:

- Take a 2-week vacation from caregiving.
- Get help from a community organization for caregiving tasks.
- Exercise 3 times a week for 30 minutes each time.

- Work on a new hobby or job idea for 5 hours a week.

Get rid of negativity

There's enough negativity in this world; you don't need to add to it by being negative toward yourself. Negative self-talk is another barrier that can get in the way of your caring for yourself and achieving your goals.

Saying things to yourself like, "I can never find the time to do the things I want," or "I can never do anything right" is counter-productive and can cause unnecessary anxiety.

Instead, try talking positively to yourself. Use the words "I can do ..." and "I'm good at..." to start your sentences. Remember, your mind is very powerful and believes what you tell it.

Identify personal barriers

Do you find it easier to take care of others than to take care of yourself? If this has been a pattern, you may have beliefs and personal barriers standing in the way of your taking care of yourself.

If that's the case, ask yourself: What good will you be to your loved one if you get sick or, even worse, if you die?

Breaking old patterns can be challenging, but it can be done. It doesn't matter what caregiving situation you're in or how long you've been in it.

The first step in removing personal barriers to caring for yourself is to identify what is in your way. Try asking yourself these questions:

1. Do I think I'm being selfish if I put my needs first?
2. Do I have trouble asking for what I need, or do I feel like a failure if I do?
3. Do I do too much because I feel as though I have to prove that I'm worthy of my loved one's affection?

Another barrier that can get in the way of proper self-care is having misconceptions about caregiving.

See if you identify with any of these statements:

- I am responsible for my mom's/dad's health.
- If I don't do it, no one will.
- If I do it right, I will get the love, attention, and respect I deserve.
- I promised my mom that I would always take care of my dad.

Beliefs or misconceptions like these can cause caregivers to continually try to do what can't be done and control what can't be controlled.

This leads to frustration and feelings of being a failure, which themselves lead to a lack of self-care. If you're not taking good care of yourself, ask yourself what barriers may be in your way.

CHAPTER 46
How Do I Find Time for ME?

When I let go of what I am, I become what I might be.
~ Lao Tzu

Life as a caregiver can be so jam-packed, you may wonder how you could ever find extra time for yourself. This is especially true for those of you who are sandwich caregivers, juggling the care of your kids with the care of a parent with Parkinson's.

Here's a ray of sunshine – caregivers who do find time for themselves end up with more energy and are better at stress management, enabling them to be better caregivers.

Most caregivers like the idea of "me time" but are convinced that they can't find it. You can! Believe it and bit by bit you will achieve it!

Here are some strategies to help you find "me time":

Schedule it

Many people use daily, weekly and monthly planners and calendars to keep track of all their work and family tasks. Choose an organizational system that works best for you, then use it to schedule "me time" every day.

Even if it's only 15 minutes, write it in your daily "to-do" list and make a commitment to making this time for yourself every day. Ideally you'll want to schedule this time early in the day to make sure other tasks don't bump you off the calendar.

If you're not used to making "me time" a priority, it may take some time to get in a habit of doing so. That's why it's so important that you schedule it and stick to it. Many professionals have said that it takes 3 weeks to build a new habit, so give yourself at least that amount of time to make this change.

Make sure you use your scheduled "me time" for something you enjoy, not for something like doing laundry or paying bills. Indulge in a nice cup of tea and a brand-new book. If you have a favorite art or craft (for me it's scrapbooking), set up a craft table and have some fun!

In addition to your daily break, schedule a larger chunk of time once a week to do something for yourself away from home. This could include a spa day, shopping, or meeting up with friends for a movie.

Learn to say "no."

This is a tough one, I know. Though you may be able to say yes to most of your loved one's requests, there may be times when you need to say no, especially if they're asking you to take on a new task that would interfere with your own personal time (which is absolutely necessary for you to keep if you want to be an effective caregiver).

If you have a hard time saying no to your loved one's request, there are a couple strategies you can try. First, you can delay your answer. For example, you could say, "I'm not sure, let me get back to you." By answering this way, you give yourself time to think about whether or not the request is something you can and/or are willing to do. You will have to practice saying no and expressing regrets if you haven't done this much before. Don't worry, the more you do it, the easier it gets.

Another way to answer a request to which you want to say no, whether it be to your care receiver or anyone else, is by saying something like, "I wish I could help but it will have to be another time." Or "I'd love to help but I just have too much going on right now."

Create a "me space"

Having a space in your home that is just for you can be a great way to get away while still being near your loved one if you need to be. This personal retreat area can be something as simple as a comfy chair in a corner or a window nook. Or, if you have the space, you can create a "woman/man cave" in a spare room or the garage.

Wherever you choose to create this personal space, make sure it's somewhere you can relax and be on your own (you may have to ask family members to respect your privacy when you're there).

Decorate it with your favorite pictures and meaningful mementos, and stock it with anything you want to have nearby for your getaway (books, crafts, music, etc.).

Delegate or share tasks

To ensure you have the best chance of "me time" throughout your caregiving journey, minimize the time you spend on tasks that don't absolutely need your personal involvement.

To do this, you will need to delegate or share tasks. For example, is there anyone in your household who could make dinner once a week? Could they do house cleaning or yard work? If you have kids, find areas with which they may be able to help. Consider making a chore schedule, with everyone in the household taking a shift.

As a caregiver you may tend to help your loved one more than they actually need. Remember to let your loved one do the things they can still do for themselves. If he or she can still fold laundry or clean a sink (even if they don't perform the task as perfectly as you'd like), let them. This will help them feel useful and also enable you to free up time.

Find shortcuts

One way to make time for yourself is to be more efficient with the time you're already using. Spend a day analyzing how you do your routine tasks to see if you could be more efficient.

For example, schedule medical appointments first thing in the morning or right after lunch to avoid long waiting room times. Instead of going into your bank to pay bills, do your banking online. Run your errands when traffic is lightest and crowds are thinner.

Another way to be more efficient is to multitask. For example, use a Bluetooth in your car to make phone calls while driving to appointments or running errands. To catch up on your favorite pre-recorded shows, watch them while you're getting your workout done on the treadmill.

If you can afford a laptop, iPad or eReader of some kind, these can be great investments for maximizing your time. You can use them while waiting for appointments, on the bus or in between errands. These devices can be used to catch up on any work you have to do, or if you're in need of some "me time," you can download your favorite books on them to save time on going to the library or bookstore.

Get unplugged

Here's a fairly easy way to make time for yourself; unplug for a bit. Almost all of us use electronic devices of some kind throughout the day, whether they are our phones, computers or TVs.

The question is, how much of that time is wisely spent? In other words, do you spend hours surfing the Internet aimlessly or reading and posting on Facebook, Twitter or Instagram? Admittedly, it's nice to have electronics when you want to multitask, but they can become dangerous time-suckers if you aren't careful.

Start paying attention to how much time you spend plugged in every day. Consider taking a break from your devices, even if it's for only 20 minutes a day.

See how it feels to be free of all electronics. You may find it easier to focus on your interactions with others, and have deeper connections with them. You may also discover that you have a lot more free time for "me time" in a day than you originally thought.

Buy time

If you can afford to buy services to help make your life less burdened, busy or chaotic, do it. This is one thing I've never heard of someone regretting.

There are so many services available that can save you time and energy; house cleaning, grocery delivery, meal delivery and yard work are just a few.

Of course, there's also the previously mentioned professional caregiving services, adult day care and elder companion services.

If you're not sure whether you want to spend the extra money on these kinds of services, consider how much of your valuable time hiring someone to do these things will save you.

To save money, consider paying a young relative or neighborhood kid to do yard work for you. You may be able to find help through local churches, Boy/Girl Scout troops or schools as well.

If you really have no extra money left at the end of each month, consider asking relatives who have offered help but who can't because they don't live nearby. Helping out financially could be an alternative way for them to contribute to your caregiving load.

If and when you choose to buy yourself some time, do yourself a favor and spend that time on YOU. Though you may be tempted to simply run errands, aim to do something meaningful as well. Choose an activity that will nourish you so that you can come back to your caregiving tasks refreshed.

CHAPTER 47
How to Minimize
Caregiver Weight Gain

Nothing tastes as great as fit feels.
~ Anthony Robbins

When I first found out that caregiver weight gain was a "thing," I was actually quite relieved. Maybe then I could blame the extra 10-15 pounds I'd been carrying around for the last couple years on my caring for Mom.

Apparently gaining 10 or even 20 pounds is very common for people while they're on a caregiving journey. The stress of it all can lead to emotional eating, stress eating, or fast eating with poor food choices.

I know I've been guilty of stress and emotional eating. Sometimes I grab junk food or overeat without thinking about it. Even though intellectually I know better, unless it's convenient and tasty (no offense to the tofu lovers out there, but sometimes I need a bit more zing to my food), I tend to cut corners in the "nutritional eating" department.

One thing that has helped me get a bit better at this has simply been paying more attention to my food choices. I've also started to pay closer attention to portion size, especially on days when I haven't been able to get in my swim workout.

Another step I've taken to ensure that I'm getting all the nutrients I need is taking a multivitamin every day.

Here are some more tips to help lessen caregiver weight gain:

- PLAN AHEAD. The easiest way to eat healthier is to prepare healthy snacks ahead of time. Chop up fresh fruit and veggies and keep them in a Ziploc bag in the fridge (or, even better, save time and buy them pre-chopped!). You can also buy nuts (e.g., walnuts, almonds, cashews), which are great, good-for-you snacks on the go. Another quick, healthy snack is air-popped popcorn.

- Eat for energy. Think of your body as a car that needs fuel. If you constantly fill your tank with junk and processed foods (a.k.a. empty calories), you can't expect your engine to perform at its best. Instead, choose foods that will keep your blood sugar stable and provide lots of energy. These include lean protein at every meal, whole grains (e.g., oats), foods high in omega-3 fatty acids (e.g., salmon) and lots of plant-based foods, including fruits, vegetables, and nuts.

- Stick to simple recipes with minimal ingredients to get meals onto your plate sooner. For example, for dinner you could pan fry a chicken breast, heat up some frozen vegetables and make 5-minute brown rice.

- When you cook, make enough for leftovers to have the next day, or freeze them for another time when you need a quick meal.

- Pay attention to what you're eating. Avoid multi-tasking during meal times so that you can really taste and enjoy your food, as well as pay attention to portion sizes.

- Get help from friends and family to prepare your snacks or bring over dinner when you feel overwhelmed.

- Don't self-medicate with alcohol. For example, it's okay to enjoy your wine, but make sure you're not using alcohol as a crutch. I am a red wine lover, but moderation is key for me to maintain a healthy weight.

- If cooking for yourself and your loved one is becoming more and more difficult, consider home-delivered meal services. Your loved one may qualify to get these paid for by a government program, so it's a good idea to look into that.

- Try pre-made nutritional shakes when you have to skip a meal.

- Don't forbid yourself to eat yummy, comforting foods like chocolate. It's okay to have this from time to time, just watch how much you eat – moderation is key.

- If you have a sweet tooth like I do, try lower fat/lower sugar alternatives like gelato instead of ice cream. In the summer, try fresh berries on top of angel food cake instead of a heavier, more calorically dense cheesecake.

- Strive to reduce high-sugar and high-fat foods from your diet, but don't eliminate all fat. Olive oil, flax seed oil, and the oil in nuts and fish such as salmon are considered healthy fats. One of my favorite "good fat'" foods is avocado. I eat one of these almost every day on my salad. Homemade guacamole is also a tasty treat!

- If you're taking medications, find out if any of them interact with the food you're eating, as they may cause weight gain. You can ask your doctor or pharmacist about this. Also check out the National Library of Medicine's MedlinePlus website for detailed info: www.nlm.nih.gov/medlineplus.

- Don't forget that exercising every day can help with maintaining weight. Just remember: you can never out-exercise a bad diet!

--- ~ ---
PART 9
TOUGH CAREGIVING
DECISIONS & ISSUES
--- ~ ---

CHAPTER 48
Decisions About Driving:
When is it Time to Take Away the Keys?

Courage is resistance to fear, mastery of fear -not absence of fear.
~ Mark Twain

Many people think that once they have been diagnosed with Parkinson's they will have to give up driving. This isn't necessarily true. Each case of Parkinson's is unique and the disease progresses at a different rate in each person.

Although driving isn't safe in the advanced stages of Parkinson's, people with milder symptoms who can control their impaired motor abilities can continue driving.

If you are the primary caregiver for someone with PD, it's important for you to know that there are several issues involved in deciding whether or not your loved one should be driving. Factors like their physical ability, legal permission, safety, and the importance of keeping their independence all play a part.

Most likely, your loved one will be able to drive safely and legally for several years, depending on their age and general physical condition. However, PD and its medications eventually affect reaction time, ability to handle multiple tasks, vision, and judgment.

If you're thinking that driving may be of concern for your loved one, a few questions you will want to ask yourself are: Do they get lost frequently? Do other drivers honk at them? Do they have trouble staying in their own lane? If so, it might be time for them to give up the keys.

If you do not feel that your loved one is safe, there are a few approaches you can take with them. First, you can take the direct approach. "Mom, do you think you should be driving anymore? It scares me to get in the car with you and I'm afraid you're going to hurt/kill someone."

Another angle would be to call your local driver's license office and express to them your concerns. They can have your loved one take a road test, which he or she will not be able to pass.

Finally, you could ask their doctor to call and have their license revoked. In extreme circumstances, you may need to disconnect the vehicle battery and take away their keys.

My mom stopped driving about 15 years after her diagnosis because it caused her to tense up and that caused her muscles to hurt. She also found her dyskinesia to be too much of an issue. She just felt safer having her husband drive.

CHAPTER 49
Convincing Your Loved One They Need Home Care

The closest thing to being cared for is to care for someone else.
~ Carson McCullers

If you've been caring for your loved one in your home for some time, or if your loved one lives alone but is no longer able to properly care for himself or herself, you may have considered getting outside help.

Considering Home Care doesn't mean you don't want to be a caregiver anymore or that you don't love your spouse or family member; as the primary caregiver, it's your *responsibility* to keep your loved one safe, healthy, and properly cared for.

Though your loved one may wish to live at home, they may not like the idea of having outside caregivers come into their house. You may need to help your loved one understand why they need help, and why this option is best for you as well.

When you talk with your loved one about the possibility of choosing Home Care, make sure you listen to their thoughts and feelings. Put yourself in their shoes – it's not easy losing independence and freedom. Be sensitive and empathetic towards them.

You might talk about burnout and how this will eventually happen to you if you don't get outside help. This will mean that you will no longer be able to care for them.

Next, explain why having some outside help could be a way to learn new things, as well as have some new company in the house for your loved one.

You might suggest a trial period so that both of you can see how and if this would be good for your situation. Remind your loved one that in the end, what helps you as the caregiver will also help them.

Your loved one may need time to accept that they need help, so be patient and give them the time and space they need to come to terms with this.

CHAPTER 50
The Dreaded Nursing Home Decision

We accept the love we think we deserve.
~ Stephen Chbosky

When Mom appointed me as POA for her care, I was both honored and afraid. Honored that she felt she could entrust *me* to make sure she got the best quality of care as possible, and scared that it might be a very hard thing to do.

This happened a few years before Mom developed dementia. Thankfully, she had the forethought to do so, because it turns out that there are many care decisions that need to be made when it comes to the later stages of Parkinson's disease.

When Mom gave me this "mission," I told her I would do my upmost to make sure she would get the best quality of care, to live the best quality of life, for as long as she possibly could. After all, Mom would have done nothing less for me.

When it comes to the nursing home discussion, this is something Mom was able to have with her family before she developed dementia. Again, this was fortunate for us, as we could then feel less stress about making this hard decision.

We (Mom, Dave (my step-dad), and us kids) made the decision together that Mom would try out a nursing home. Things were just getting too overwhelming for Dave; his health was going downhill and none of us was in the position to house my mom, let alone give her the round-the-clock care that she needed.

Though it certainly wasn't an easy decision for any of us, over time we have seen that choosing to be in a nursing home was the best thing for Mom.

Most people cringe at the thought of moving their loved one into a nursing home. This is totally understandable, given most of their not-so-wonderful reputations. However, there may come a point in your caregiving journey when your loved one's needs exceed the care you can give them and it becomes in their best interest to move them into a long-term care facility.

Of course, every situation is different, so there's no definite answer as to whether or not – or when – you should move your loved one into a nursing home.

If you're having a hard time with the nursing home decision, there are a few things you should remember. First, placing your loved one in a nursing home isn't mean or selfish. As was said before, it can be in the best interest of your loved one. Second, remember that it's the disease making it necessary for you to do this, NOT you failing at caregiving.

Finally, know that you don't have to make this decision alone. Talking it over with your loved one's doctor, a minister, or a social worker can help you work through various issues in the decision-making process. This will take the burden off you and allow you to feel less alone in the process.

One of the positives that can come from placing your loved one in a nursing home is connection. Because you no longer have to take care of your loved one's physical needs, you can focus on loving them and connecting with them in more emotional ways.

Delaying nursing home placement

Here's a little "P.S." to this discussion. If you're not sure whether the timing is right or if you want to delay placing your loved one in a nursing home, you may want to try Adult Day Care.

As mentioned in a previous chapter, Adult Day Care can give you and your family respite during the day while allowing your loved one to have access to the services and care they need. This may be a great solution until your loved one's care needs increase.

CHAPTER 51
Keeping the Peace in the Family

There are two ways of spreading light –
to be the candle or the mirror that reflects it.
~ Edith Wharton

Things can get a bit tricky with family as you get further down the road with Parkinson's. As with any chronic illness, when a loved one starts to show signs of needing more care, there are many issues for family members to discuss and numerous important decisions that need to be made.

Sometimes the severity of these decisions and their potential implications can cause very heated discussions within a family.

Depending on how big your family is, and how many people want to be involved in the caregiving process (even if it's not hands on), having family meetings to discuss your loved one's care needs can be both practical and helpful.

Before you have these meetings, it's important to keep a few things in mind. First, know that it's not uncommon for family members to disagree over how a loved one should be cared for. Even the most harmonious siblings can become divided on various topics relating to their parents' care.

The good news is that peace is possible throughout the process.

Try these strategies to help keep the peace when discussing your loved one's care needs with family:

Plan ahead

Before you have your family meeting, you'll want to choose the right place for it. Whether it's physically in the same room or on a conference call using Skype or FaceTime, it's important that every member feels welcome and comfortable.

The next thing you'll want to do is have a few key points written down that you want to cover during the conversation. If applicable, bring an up-to-date medical report on your loved one, as well as a list of your loved one's wants and needs with regards to care and support from the family.

Some questions you may want to discuss are where your loved one will live (e.g., in their home, with another family member, in assisted living), how much their care will cost and how that cost will be covered, how much time each family member has to visit or care for your loved one, and what the primary caregiver needs in terms of assistance and support from the family.

Accept that not everyone may want to be involved

Understand that not everyone in your family may want to be involved in the planning of your loved one's care. Whatever their reasons for wanting to be excluded, it's important to respect their decision. You don't have to agree with it, but it's helpful to try to be understanding. If you let resentment build up, it won't be good for anyone.

Consider outside help

Every family member should be allowed to express his or her thoughts and feelings without being criticized or interrupted. If you happen to be in one of those families that likes to talk over or yell and fight with each other, you may want to think about asking an objective third party to sit in on the meeting and help facilitate the conversation. A few people you could consider are a family friend, a social worker, or a pastor.

Identify caregiving roles and responsibilities

The roles and responsibilities of your family members will depend on their individual relationship with your loved one, how much time they have to give, and where they live.

For example, if your sister lives far away from your loved one, she won't be able to give hands-on care, but she may be able to take charge of setting up appointments or managing finances.

Accept when things don't go perfectly

Don't expect to solve every problem in one meeting. It's inevitable that some questions will go answered and not all plans will work out the way you thought they would. If you can accept the fact that sometimes your family will disagree or fight, it will allow you to stay calm and steer the conversation back to the problem at hand if things get off track.

Get organized and keep others in the loop

When it comes to keeping peace in a family, I've found that the best offense is defense. If you keep members informed and updated about your loved one's status and care, a lot of problems and confusion can be avoided.

Come up with a strategy for keeping family members informed. If there are any unexpected changes or there's an emergency, consider setting up a phone tree to spread the word.

After you have a family meeting, consider writing down a summary of what you talked about, what decisions were made, etc., and emailing it to all family members.

Also, because family meetings are most effective if they are held on a regular basis, make a tentative schedule for when the family should gather again to re-evaluate a loved one's care.

CHAPTER 52
Parkinson's & Dementia:
Caregiving for a Double Diagnosis

*In the depth of winter, I finally learned that within me
there lay an invincible summer.*
~ Albert Camus

After having had Parkinson's for 20 years, it wasn't a huge surprise for my family to learn that Mom had started developing dementia as well. I had read the statistics in numerous places – as many as 50 to 80 percent of people with Parkinson's disease could eventually experience dementia.

In addition to this statistic, studies have found that those who do develop dementia do so between 10 and 15 years after their original Parkinson's diagnosis. I guess Mom beat the odds there.

It's tough when a loved one is diagnosed with Parkinson's, and even more so when you get a double diagnosis of dementia.

Parkinson's dementia is more difficult on caregivers than some of the other types of dementia like Alzheimer's, because of the added impact of motor loss in Parkinson's. Though the disease is progressive, it can last many years, so it's very important to learn the best ways to care for your loved one, as well as yourself, in order to continue providing care for many years.

To begin, it's a good idea to be educated about Parkinson's dementia:

Who gets Parkinson's dementia?

The people with Parkinson's who have the most risk of developing dementia are those who have hallucinations, mild cognitive impairment (MCI), excessive daytime sleepiness, and/or more severe motor control problems. There's also a higher incidence of Parkinson's dementia in men than in women.

*Note: Sometimes dementia in a person with Parkinson's disease can be caused by Vitamin B12 deficiency, depression, or thyroid dysfunction, so make sure your loved one's doctor investigates their symptoms thoroughly.

How is Parkinson's dementia different from Alzheimer's?

These are some symptoms of Parkinson's dementia that may vary from those of Alzheimer's and other dementias. With Parkinson's disease dementia (PDD), people usually have major problems with attention, have a hard time making decisions, experience challenges with planning and reasoning, have slow thought processes, and encounter difficulties with memory retrieval.

In Alzheimer's disease, there is a great loss of memory and intellectual abilities. The memory problem is more often one of storing memories as opposed to retrieving them, as in PDD. People with PDD may also have more insight into the fact that they have a memory problem than do people with Alzheimer's disease.

In cases where doctors determine that Parkinson's disease is the cause of dementia, the official diagnosis would be *Dementia Due to Parkinson's disease*.

What are the symptoms of Parkinson's dementia?

• Changes in memory, concentration, and judgment
• Difficulty concentrating, slowed thinking
• Trouble completing tasks
• Trouble shifting attention from task to task
• Trouble interpreting visual information and depth perception
• Muffled speech and difficulty with word finding
• Visual hallucinations

- Delusions, especially paranoid ideas
- Depression and lack of motivation
- Irritability/moodiness and anxiety
- Disorientation
- Sleep disturbances, including excessive daytime drowsiness and rapid eye movement (REM) sleep disorder

How to care for someone with Parkinson's dementia

To help your loved one in the early stages of dementia, encourage them to do the following:

- Stay mentally active (card games, board games, etc.)
- Stay physically active (walking, stretching, etc.)
- Do things they enjoy (hobbies, shopping with you, etc.)
- Stay socially engaged
- Stay positive
- Get enough sleep
- Relax

Try these strategies to make caregiving tasks easier:

- Embrace their reality. It's okay to tell little fibs to your loved one (e.g. that their spouse is still alive, even if he or she isn't), as this will keep them happier.
- Stay on schedule (to reduce confusion).
- Make sure all living areas are well lit to prevent falls.
- Remove anything (or anyone) that could over-stimulate your loved one.
- Make your loved one's living environment "wander-proof."
- If your loved one gets agitated, try to determine the source. Use distraction and redirection if you can't calm them down.

- Keep lots of snacks handy as people with dementia often have a hard time explaining what they want.
- Play your loved one's favorite music whenever you can.
- Learn CPR and the Heimlich maneuver.
- Care for yourself by connecting with others and getting respite.

You may find attending a support group for Alzheimer's in addition to attending one for Parkinson's to be helpful in caring for the dementia side of things.

If you find getting out of the house is hard, there are online support groups and forums (see the appendix at the end of this book for a list) that can help you cope with your daily challenges without your having to leave your loved one's side.

Remember, the more help and support you can get, the longer you'll be able to care for your loved one and the better caregiver you'll be.

CHAPTER 53
Grieving While Your Loved One is Still Alive

It takes strength to make your way through grief,
to grab hold of your life and let it pull you forward.
~ Patti Davis

I've been trying to keep it together for a long time. Trying so hard not to say good-bye to Mom because my mind keeps saying, "She's still here! She's not gone yet!" I guess a part of me thinks that if I say good-bye, it will actually make her gone. That part just sucks the life out of me.

For those who have never experienced dementia in their lives, it's tough to explain. I have some very kind and well-wishing friends who say that they're sorry about my mom having dementia, but that I should at least be thankful she's still alive. I know they're right to some extent, but it's still hard and I know they can't fully understand what I'm going through.

Though technically she's still here, Mom's not the same Mom I used to know. She hasn't been for quite some time. She's a new mom whom I've been getting used to, so much so that sometimes I forget the old Mom.

I've mourned many losses along her dementia journey, and I know that with this kind of caregiving, it's normal to experience a series of losses before the final good-bye.

Grieving a loved one while they're still alive applies to all kinds of caregiving situations. Those of you who are saying good-bye to a loved one with an illness that causes memory loss like Parkinson's dementia will especially relate.

You may find it weird talking about grieving when someone hasn't actually died yet, but psychologists say that grieving doesn't require a loss of life. They say that whether or not a person is still alive doesn't matter; the emotional process of grieving is the same.

If you're experiencing grief while caring for a loved one, there are some ways to make life a bit easier.

Here are some key tips to help you in the grieving process:

- Be kind to yourself. Recognize that grieving can take a toll on your physical and emotional health. Allow yourself to take guilt-free breaks, be emotional when you need to be, and treat yourself to experiences that nourish your mind and soul.

- Give yourself permission to live your life. This has been a tough one for me, as I have felt for a long time that my life needed to be on hold until my caregiving duties were done and Mom was gone. Over time I have come to realize that Mom would always want me to be happy and wouldn't want me to miss out on all that life has to offer.

- Slow down. Be present. Breathe. Caring for someone with dementia demands that you do these things.

- Reach out; confide in other caregivers or support groups who know and understand what you're going through.

- Celebrate and cherish the memories you have with your loved one. Consider putting together an album (complete with photos and journal entries) commemorating their life story.

- Get help from hospice care workers. They are trained to help those who have a life expectancy of less than 6 to 12 months, and also work with families to help process grief.

--- ~ ---

--- ~ ---

APPENDIX

--- ~ ---

Caregiver Resources

Caregiver Organizations

The National Alliance for Caregiving:
www.caregiving.org

Caregiver Action Network USA:
www.caregiveraction.org

Family Caregiver Alliance
www.caregiver.org

Financial Resources

If you live in the U.S.:

www.payingforseniorcare.com

If you live in Canada:

www.aplaceformom.com/canada/how-to-pay-for-senior-housing

If you live in Australia:

www.humanservices.gov.au/customer/subjects/payments-older-
australians

If you live in the U.K.:

www.carehome.co.uk

www.housingcare.org/elderly-uk-nursing-homes.aspx

www.careuk.com/care-homes/

Housing Help

For housing help in the U.S.:

www.aplaceformom.com

For housing help in the U.K.:

www.ageuk.org.uk/home-and-care/housing-choices

For housing help in Canada:

www.aplaceformom.com/canada

For housing help in Australia:

www.seniorshousingonline.com.au

Online Caregiver Courses

For all types of caregiving:

www.homesweethomecareinc.com/cargiving-training-education/family-caregiver-trainin

www.seniorsresourceguide.com/directories/National/CaregiverClasses/index.html

www.caregiverlist.com/caregiver-training-center

For Alzheimer's and dementia caregiving:

www.alz.org/care/alzheimers-dementia-care-training-certification.asp

www.oregoncarepartners.com/classes/online

Online Forums/Support Groups

www.allaboutparkinsons.com/forum

www.parkinsons.org.uk/forum/carers-friends-and-family

www.caring.com/support-groups

www.caregiver.com/regionalresources

www.agingcare.com/Caregiver-Forum

Helpful Gadgets for
People With Parkinson's

** This section has been copied from our first book, "Everything You Need to Know About Parkinson's Disease" because we feel that it can help caregivers as much as it can help people with Parkinson's. We've added a few more gadgets to the list to make it even more helpful.

Here are our top gadget recommendations for people with Parkinson's:

Grabbers and Reachers

Even though these aren't very high-tech, they can be extremely useful for day-to-day living. Having one of these long, thin tools to act as a secure hand that picks up stuff from the ground can help people with Parkinson's keep their independence and also help reduce the risk of falling.

LaserCane

The LaserCane is a great tool to help people with Parkinson's walk smoothly. As you take your normal steps, the cane projects a bright red line across your path. This line acts as a visual cue to help break freezing episodes and increase stride length.

The LaserCane is perfect for those seeking minor walking support with freeze-reduction technology. You can find out more about the LaserCane here: www.ustep.com/cane.htm

Medical Alert System

There are many options out there for systems that can alert someone if you're having an emergency at home. One system that has received a lot of attention is *The CareLine Home Safety Telephone System*. It is an all-in-one communications center that includes a corded base and cordless handset with large-text display, large amber-backlit buttons, and audio boost.

Other features include the answering machine's ability to play back messages in slow mode to make them easier to understand and voice dialing, which allows a person to call up to 50 numbers set up on the system.

The best feature is the portable and rechargeable CareLine pendant. This pendant acts like a mini-cordless phone that an older person can wear around their neck. It comes with two programmable buttons, so you could program one to call you or a caregiver, and the other to call 911.

Fall Detectors

If your loved one has problems with balance or extra-fragile bones, fall detectors are very important.

Some medical alert systems also come with automatic fall detection, which senses when an elderly person has fallen down. Though these types of systems usually cost more, they can be worth it, especially in certain situations.

If a person falls and is unresponsive, the medical alert system will notify the call center automatically. In addition, the latest technology provides gyroscopes that can sense dramatic changes in position and alert backup, even if the person is not conscious.

Handheld Massagers

Pain often accompanies Parkinson's disease, so it's important to learn ways to manage or relieve it. Whether it be in the neck, shoulder, or leg, these types of pain can all be helped by massage. If you find going to a registered massage therapist to be too costly, handheld massagers are a great alternative. There are many different kinds, ranging from $10 to

$200. Check your local drug or department store. You can also find many options online.

Big Button Cell Phone

If you've been intimidated by smartphones, you don't have to worry. There are other phones, like the Jitterbug 5 from Samsung, that serve many purposes, including acting as a medical alert system.

Some of the key features of this phone are:

- Big buttons with large, legible numbers to make dialing easy
- Backlit keypad to assist visibility in low-light areas
- Bright-colored screen so you can easily see phone numbers, text messages, and photos
- Hearing aid compatible (M4/T4 rating) with a powerful speaker so that conversations are loud and clear

Automatic Pill Reminders

If you know anything about Parkinson's medications, you know how important it is that you take them as prescribed. Being on time is especially important; to help you do this, there are various options on the market for pill reminders.

One of the more basic types of pill reminders is a pillbox that is labeled according to the days of the week. These kinds of reminders need to be filled accurately at the beginning of the week, but after that the pills are easy to find and take.

Another, newer method of medication packaging is the blister or bubble pack. You may have seen these in the hospital; the packs are prepared by the pharmacy, and each pack contains one day's worth of pills, or pills to be taken at a certain time (i.e., breakfast or dinner).

There are also pill boxes that come with alarms. Or, if you prefer, you can buy a digital watch with multiple alarms so that you can be reminded throughout the day to take your meds.

Skype

If you have never heard of Skype, it's an awesome FREE online service that can make such a difference in the lives of family and friends.

With a simple download to your computer, iPad, tablet, or smartphone, this service allows you to see and talk to another person in real time.

I set up Skype for my mom 5 years ago on her computer and tablet and we've been using it ever since. It's been a real Godsend during the times we've had to be apart.

ALSO BY LIANNA MARIE

Everything You Need to Know About Parkinson's Disease

199 Helpful Tips for People With Parkinson's –
Tips, Advice & Stories That Make Living with Parkinson's Easier

A Helpful Guide for Parkinson's Caregivers –
15 Vital Tips to Help You Care for the Person You Know or Love

67 Practical Tips for People with Parkinson's –
Make Your Life Easier, Happier, and More Productive

What You Need to Know About Pain and Parkinson's –
A Simple Guide to Relieving Parkinson's Related Aches and Pains

Find these books and more at:
www.allaboutparkinsons.com

Made in the USA
San Bernardino, CA
17 May 2020